Medicine of the Person

of related interest

Anthropological Approaches to Psychological Medicine
Crossing Bridges
Edited by Vieda Skultans and John Cox
ISBN 1 85302 708 1 pb
ISBN 1 85302 707 3 hb

Health, the Individual, and Integrated Medicine
Revisiting an Aesthetic of Health Care
David Aldridge
ISBN 1 84310 232 3

Making Sense of Spirituality in Nursing and Health Care Practice
An Interactive Approach
Second Edition
Wilfred McSherry
Foreword by Keith Cash
ISBN 1 84310 365 6

Talking about Spirituality in Health Care Practice
A Resource for the Multi-Professional Health Care Team
Gillian White
ISBN 1 84310 305 2

Spirituality in Health Care Contexts
Edited by Helen Orchard
Foreword by Julia Neuberger
ISBN 1 85302 969 6

Spirituality and Mental Health Care
Rediscovering a 'Forgotten' Dimension
John Swinton
ISBN 1 85302 804 5

Working Relationships
Spirituality in Human Service and Organisational Life
Neil Pembroke
ISBN 1 84310 252 8

Passionate Medicine
Making the Transition from Conventional Medicine to Homeopathy
Edited by Robin Shohet
ISBN 1 84310 298 6

Medicine of the Person

Faith, Science and Values in Health Care Provision

Edited by John Cox, Alastair V. Campbell and Bill (K.W.M.) Fulford

Foreword by Julia Neuberger

Jessica Kingsley Publishers
London and Philadelphia

First published in 2007
by Jessica Kingsley Publishers
116 Pentonville Road
London N1 9JB, UK
and
400 Market Street, Suite 400
Philadelphia, PA 19106, USA

www.jkp.com

Library of Congress Cataloging in Publication Data
A CIP catalog record for this book is available from the Library of Congress

British Library Cataloguing in Publication Data
A CIP catalogue record for this book is available from the British Library

ISBN-13: 978 1 84310 397 4
ISBN-10: 1 84310 397 4

Printed and bound in Great Britain by
Athenaeum Press, Gateshead, Tyne and Wear

CONTENTS

PART 2 – Faith Traditions and Medicine of the Person

PART 3 – Medicine of the Person in Contemporary Practice

FOREWORD

This fascinating volume tries to get to grips with the science/religion debate. In the footsteps of the great Christian doctor, Paul Tournier, it tries to argue that we need both science and faith – or at least values. And our varying faiths, cultures and values need addressing within the health care system. So health care professionals need to think beyond the wholly clinical and scientific approach, and look instead to a more personal interaction. Nurses need to recognize the person's culture, faith and values as well as their clinical needs in terms of drugs and cleanliness. Doctors need to think about how a Hindu or a Jew perceives illness, and set it within a context they understand, rather than simply talking in terms of a particular diagnosis. And the importance of recognizing the individual's spirituality can never be overstated.

So far, so good. Interesting, but not perhaps wholly surprising. Yet what all the authors argue for is a highly individualized approach to patients that makes much of modern medicine look distinctly poor quality. The mass approach of much modern care, with a clinical team providing care to a whole cohort of patients, sits decidedly uncomfortably with an approach that seeks to understand how the patient views his or her own illness, what illness means to them, and how their own tradition views medicine and the saving of life. A Jew is brought up to believe that one must do everything in one's power to save life; one's own as well as others'. A Hindu takes a different view, meanwhile seeing psychosis in very different terms from Jews, Christians and Muslims. We need to understand how the different faiths view suffering, how they understand pain, how they approach mental distress, and what they have to say to those whose prognosis is one of an early death. Yet our health services prefer to produce protocols telling staff how patients with particular conditions should be treated, rather than how people of different backgrounds and views should helped.

This volume is timely, and impressive. Indirectly, it is asking those who run our National Health Service, and other health services around the world, what they will do to put the personal back into health care. It ought to be required reading for politicians, civil servants and managers who run health services, so that they can reflect on the essential quality of the personal relationship in achieving a good outcome. Nature versus nurture is not the question: better outcomes for those who have a religious faith may be one of the underlying issues, but the real question is whether modern health services can be sufficiently individualistic, as well as scientifically sound, to make people feel cared for as well as treated clinically the best way possible. If they can, then the dynamic interpersonal encounter of health professional and patient has been achieved, to everyone's benefit. If not, then the atmosphere of health care for the twenty-first century will be one of reductionist scientism, with very little holistic care for the patients who need it more than anything else.

This volume makes a powerful case, pushing a cause with which I have been concerned for my entire adult life. I hope that those who need to read it and inwardly digest will do so, and that it will have the influence it so obviously deserves.

Julia Neuberger

PREFACE

This book was triggered when, as a novice medical student in Oxford, I first read Dr Paul Tournier's *Doctor's Casebook in the Light of the Bible*. At that time I was searching for a bridge between the basic sciences and the Christian faith tradition.

Much later, at a meeting of the International Medicine of the Person Group in Prague, 1993, I was intrigued by the memories and wholesome relationships of these continental doctors and their families. The 'medicine of the person' as experienced on that occasion was indeed an idea larger than that small cohesive group of fellow travellers who were well aware of the risks of a health care devoid of ethics and without sustaining compassion.

Medicine of the person is not, however, a specialist therapy nor is it psychosomatic medicine but rather an overall attitude to health care provision, restricted only by any lack of interpersonal sensitivity in the care-giver.

I never met Paul Tournier, but have read his books and talked with many doctors and their families who knew him personally. His approach to general practice in Geneva was profoundly influenced by his Christian faith. He was an orphan; his father died when he was two months old, and his mother when he was aged six. He was brought up by an uncle and aunt, and supported also by other family members and friends. Undoubtedly he was a shy, withdrawn child, almost a loner.

The emotional impact of his contact with the Oxford Group Movement was therefore a profound experience. This shy, young doctor was exposed to interpersonal dialogue and to the risk of self-exposure. It was at that time that he first started a practice, which continued to the end of his life, of a period of 'quiet time' each day. He described this as a mixture of self-reflection, musing about the day ahead and constant reflection on Bible passages. This change from an intellectual understanding of faith to a personal experience influenced his approach to medical practice. He officially informed his patients who came to him in private practice that he would in future be providing a therapy within a broader perspective that would include body, mind and spirit.

He had a sharp intellect and was well aware of the developments in scientific medicine at that time and the insights of psychoanalysis.

Medicine of the person as practised by Tournier and his colleagues gives equal attention to spiritual meanings and to scientific and psychological perspectives. This approach to health care provision is a core requirement for the provision of integrative healing and health in the contemporary world.

The contributors to this book are from different faith traditions and were each asked to illustrate facets of this approach from a scientific, faith and values perspective. Paul Tournier was a Christian, but he was very open to the beliefs of others, which could influence the understanding of health and wholeness. We hope that what these international contributors say and how they say it will stir readers to regard themselves, whether healers or healed, as persons in relationship with others; a relationship which is 'I–Thou' and therefore spiritual in the sense understood by Martin Buber.

Experiencing the enrichment of this healing approach has enlarged my own world view. Karin, my wife, was suddenly struck down by a rare brain disorder (neuro-sarcoidosis), so that she could no longer climb the hills in Cumbria. We were back at the edges of personal meanings, dusting off spiritual insights provided by the Christian community and biblical reflection, and aware that a multi-layered (axial) medical diagnosis was a crucial matter of life and death. Medicine of the person, combining prednisolone with prayer, and considering recovery strategies as well as family worries, was essential to health and wholeness. Karin can again climb hills.

'Medicine of the person' is humanistic, but it is more than that. It assumes an understanding of the economy and dynamic of the surface and depth of human experience. It touches the depth like a mutative metaphor yet is also intensely practical and pragmatic, and can be evaluated using scientific method, for example the narrative approach.

Medicine of the person maintains the morale of the doctor and the compliance of the patient and in this respect could be cost effective. In a modern context it assumes a fully functional multi-professional team that has learnt to relate to each other and to service users in an integrative way.

This book is deliberately framed within a multi-faith context. All the major world religions have as core components caring and love and going out to others. They also, at their best, can sustain professional altruism and provide explanation and solace at times of turbulence and suffering.

For Tournier and for those who reflect his initial inspiration, including the contributors to this book, medicine of the person is an encounter that requires a constant holding together of body, mind and spirit.

John Cox

ACKNOWLEDGEMENTS

It was the leaders of the Student Christian Movement and the John Wesley Society in Oxford who first encouraged John Cox to read Paul Tournier's *Doctor's Casebook in the Light of the Bible*.

The Conference held at Keele University in 1998 on 'Whole Person Medicine – the contribution of Paul Tournier' was supported by the School of Postgraduate Medicine and the John Young Foundation. Sheila Young gave us much practical help. Alastair V. Campbell, Bill Fulford, John Cox, John Clark, Thierry Collaud, Bernard Rüedi and Andrew Sims were speakers. Gordon Mursell gave an organ recital in Keele chapel and Graham Patrick led the meditation.

Karin Cox has helped us with suggestions for contributors and by encouraging the Editors.

We would like to thank the contributors and our publishers, Jessica Kingsley and Stephen Jones, for lively correspondence as well as much patience.

The idea for this book would not have germinated without the inspiration of the International and British Groups of Medicine of the Person. We acknowledge our particular thanks to all past, present and future attendees at these special meetings with their blend of faith, science and friendship. In particular we acknowledge John Clark for making available his many presentations about Paul Tournier, and for help with the bibliography. Thanks also to Bernard and Madeleine Rüedi who encouraged us to continue this particular 'Adventure of Living'.

CHAPTER I

INTRODUCTION: AT THE HEART OF HEALING

Bill (K.W.M.) Fulford, Alastair V. Campbell and John Cox

This book engages with the need to integrate the scientific basis of health care more fully with the spiritual and religious beliefs of services users and health professionals, and with the faith traditions within which these beliefs arise. Ethics is now well established as an important part of health care practice. But the growth of ethics itself, as we go on to describe in more detail, is among the factors that have led to a renewed recognition that good clinical care depends also on a wider understanding of the spiritual dimensions of health.

The flowering of scientific medicine in the twentieth century was accompanied by a progressive alienation of faith and healing. Many came to feel that medicine, in building successfully on the objective sciences, should hold itself aloof from the subjective values and beliefs of the faith traditions. It is particularly to be welcomed, therefore, that as we enter the twenty-first century there should have been a resurgence of interest in the spiritual aspects of health care. There is a growing academic literature here (e.g. Bhugra 1996; Culliford 2002; Editorial 2004; and Fulford 1996). There are also, importantly, a number of practical initiatives in policy and service delivery. In the UK's National Health Service (NHS), for example, recent reforms have included national policies aimed directly at restoring the spiritual dimension of health care (Department of Health 2003a; and Department of Health, 2003b). These developments moreover are perceived, now, not as being in opposition to science and technology but rather as supporting the delivery of care that is both evidence-based and, at the same time, closely focused on the values – the particular needs, wishes and expectations – of individual patients and their families in our increasingly multi-faith society (see e.g. Cox 1996;

National Framework of Values for Mental Health; Department of Health 2004; Department of Health 2005; and Fulford 2004, pp.205–234).

A greater understanding of the faith traditions, therefore, and of how these support and complement scientifically-based medicine as resources for healing, is urgently needed at the present time. And this is exactly where 'medicine of the person' comes in. For the defining characteristic of medicine of the person, is, precisely, that it focuses equally on the spiritual aspects of health care as on the scientific.

What is medicine of the person?

We set out and explore key aspects of medicine of the person in the four chapters making up Part 1 of the book. First, in Chapter 2, the Swiss psychiatrist and psychotherapist Hans-Rudolf Pfeifer and the British psychiatrist John Cox set the scene with an account of medicine of the person as it arose originally in post-World War II Europe, particularly through the work of Paul Tournier. As Pfeifer and Cox describe, Tournier was a General Practitioner, or family doctor, who worked in Geneva from 1925 until his death in 1986. He read widely in psychiatry and psychotherapy and he regularly met psychoanalysts (notably Alphonse Mader and Aloys von Orelli) and theologians (such as Emil Brunner) working at that time in Switzerland. He also travelled extensively in Europe, including several visits to Greece; in North America; and, later in his life, in Japan and South Africa. In the course of his lifetime, he wrote over 20 books. Although now mostly out of print, these had a considerable influence, particularly within the Christian tradition in European health care, and Tournier's ideas have subsequently been further developed through the work of the International Group for Medicine of the Person and the Paul Tournier Association (which Pfeifer helped to establish).

Though not formally trained in theology, psychotherapy or psychiatry, Tournier's wide reading in these subjects, his travels and his regular meetings with doctors, theologians and others who shared his concerns and from whom he absorbed attitudes and insights that made sense to him, gave him the basis for a theoretically well-informed but also practically focused approach to his work. This is why his books appealed not only to a medical but also to a more general readership, and particularly to those looking for a bridge between routine medical practice and Christian reflection.

Tournier, like others before him and since, regarded the professional relationship as being of paramount importance. But he added to this insight, as a unique feature of medicine of the person, the belief that for the professional relationship to be fully developed a doctor needed to understand a patient's problems equally from a faith and from a science perspective. This central theme of Tournier's work comes through clearly in his first book *Médicine de la Personne*, first published in 1940, and later books, especially *A Doctor's Case Book in the Light of the Bible* (1954) and *The Meaning of Persons* (1957). Through these and many other books Tournier argued that it was the meeting, the relationship, between the doctor and the patient, illuminated equally by faith and by science, that held the seeds of therapy and produced healing of body, mind and spirit.

The twin pillars of medicine of the person, science and faith, are the topics respectively of the next two chapters in Part 1. As noted earlier, there is a growing literature on the relationship between science and faith in medicine. Here the Swiss endocrinologist Bernard Rüedi (Chapter 3) and the British lay reader and Paul Tournier expert John Clark (Chapter 4) illustrate the ways in which science and faith respectively come together specifically in the central place of the person in Tournier's understanding of the relationship between patient and doctor – the person of the patient, and, importantly, the person of the doctor.

That the 'person' in medicine of the person includes the person of the doctor (or more widely of the health professional) as well as that of the patient, is itself important for contemporary practice. In our current concern to promote the interests of patients, we have tended to neglect those of professionals; patient-centred care has come to have an exclusive rather than inclusive meaning; and patients' rights have come to be emphasized at the expense of those of professionals. Rüedi (Chapter 3), by contrast, shows how the concept of the person in contemporary medicine of the person has an extended role, involving teamwork and relationships, and hence as being considerably wider than the doctor–patient dyad on which, consistently with the practice of his day, Tournier himself focused. Much of Clark's chapter (Chapter 4), by contrast, is concerned with the links between Tournier's work and biblical scholarship and meditation. In setting out these links, Clark shows how, in medicine of the person, these ostensibly impersonal and academic activities, of biblical scholarship and meditation, are directly harnessed to the healing process with individual people through the skills of good communication. Medicine of the person, in Tournier's powerful image, has two hands joined together as in prayer, a hand of scientific competence and a hand of personal communication.

Medicine of the person, ethics and values

This book is no mere exegesis of Tournier's work, however. It seeks rather to contribute to the development and elaboration of his person-centred approach in a modern context. The concluding chapter (Chapter 5) of Part 1 of the book, by the British radical Christian thinker Martin Conway, illustrates this point directly. Values and ethics, which in Tournier's day had little to contribute to person-centred care, are now of central significance. But as Conway shows, this increases rather than reduces the importance of the faith traditions in delivering care which, although science-based, is also genuinely patient-centred.

When Tournier was writing his influential books, the field of medical ethics was a profession-dominated and somewhat paternalistic discipline. Although guided by such high principles as those embodied in the Hippocratic oath, medical ethics often amounted in practice to little more than 'hints and tips' from senior practitioners and simplistic rules about professional behaviour. Nowadays, by contrast, medical ethics, as part of the wider field of health care ethics, has grown into a full academic subject, with a range of textbooks and academic journals to support its further development.

In practice, modern medical ethics is perhaps at risk of becoming excessively legalistic (Fulford, Thornton and Graham, 2006). But the *aims* of contemporary medical ethics are closely compatible with those endorsed by Tournier, namely to produce a 'reflective practitioner', a practitioner capable of working in an interdisciplinary way, a way that is also intellectually honest and patient-focused, and that recognizes and comes to grips with the unique position of medical practice, balanced as it is between the sciences and the humanities. And these aims of modern medical ethics are as urgently practical now as they were in Tournier's day. In all the current enthusiasm for evidence-based practice, it has become even more important to stress that medicine is an art as well as a science, and that much of the therapeutic potential of medical practice rests not on technique but, as Tournier also emphasized, on relationships. How pleased Tournier would have been, then, to see these insights restored to the heart of medical practice in the new medical ethics!

Conway's point, though, in Chapter 5 is that without a faith tradition, medical ethics, notwithstanding the enrichment of its theoretical base over the four decades since Tournier wrote his books, fails to go deep enough to meet the needs of patients or, indeed, practitioners in modern health care. Theologians, it is true, were early on the scene in medical ethics, with writers like Paul Ramsey (1970) and Richard McCormick (1981) in the USA, and Bernard Haering (1972) and Alastair V. Campbell (1975) in Europe. But soon the philosophers were to take over and for some time 'principlism' (as in Beauchamp and Childress 1994) and consequentialism (as in Singer 1993) came to dominate. The last ten years, it is also true, have seen something of a reaction to the often over-intellectualist and impersonal formulations of philosophical ethics. There has been a huge revival of interest in narrative ethics, for example, and in virtue ethics and feminist ethics, all of which demand a greater emphasis on context, on character, and on the importance of emotional as well as intellectual factors (Dickenson and Fulford 2000). A variety of other practical tools have also been developed for bringing values and evidence together in health care. Some of these, like health economics (Brown, Brown and Sharma 2005) and decision-theory (Hunink *et al.* 2001), are impersonal in approach. Others, like values-based practice (Fulford 2004, pp.205–234; Woodbridge and Fulford 2003), start from and make central the values of the individual, of the individual patient and of the individual practitioner, in an approach to health care decision-making that is close indeed to the central themes of Tournier's medicine of the person.

However, Conway's point is that these developments in ethics and value theory, although entirely compatible with and indeed complementing the faith traditions in medicine, are no substitute for them. In this new atmosphere, then, Tournier's writings on faith, spirituality and the wholeness of persons, which would have been regarded by some philosophical ethicists no less than by some scientifically minded doctors as at best irrelevant and at worst dangerously partisan, could now make an essential contribution to the new and more person-centred approach in health care.

From one faith to many?

Conway's chapter, then, shows how values and medical ethics, although hardly invented in Tournier's day and certainly not addressed in his work, are nonetheless important partners to medicine of the person in a contemporary context. With the chapters in Part 2 of the book, however, we turn to an aspect of modern health care practice that, at first glance at least, may seem to be incompatible with the insights of medicine of the person, at least as derived by Tournier, namely that, whereas Tournier worked in a predominantly Christian context, modern health care in many countries is set in contexts that are strongly multi-faith in orientation.

The importance of the Christian faith to Tournier is undeniable. All his books provide the reader with a strong sense of his Christian beliefs and spirituality, and in particular, as Clark's work (in Chapter 4) emphasizes, the value he attached to daily reflection on the Bible as a source of inspiration and as a guide to increased understanding of his patients' needs. There were theological debates raging in Europe and America at the time, but Tournier, from his writings at least, seems to have been largely insulated from them. Since the German theologian Dietrich Bonhoeffer's challenging and mysterious last writings (written prior to his execution by the Nazis) about the 'man come of age' (Bonhoeffer 1959), theologians were grappling with the puzzle of how, in a seemingly secular age, religious language could make any sense to their contemporaries. Bonhoeffer's contemporary, the systematic theologian, Paul Tillich – like Tournier strongly influenced by the writings of the Austrian psychoanalyst, Carl Jung – seemed to offer a way through the problem by stressing the inherently symbolic character of religious language (Tillich 1953). But such intellectual solutions, contrary to the tenets of Medicine of the Person, led to a more secularized approach to pastoral care and counselling. No longer were appeals to biblical texts, or advice based on biblical teaching, seen to be adequate. Instead, 'non-directiveness' or 'client-centredness' became the norm, with religious counselling following the teachings of the guru of non-directive counselling, the American psychologist and psychotherapist, Carl Rogers (1961).

Tournier, it is important to be clear, could not have accepted this collapsing of theology into psychological language and of spiritual guidance into non-directive counselling, since he believed that the insights of the Bible offered important challenges to the society of his day. For example, in his book *Guilt and Grace* (1962) he was at pains to distinguish between guilt as pathology and guilt as part of what it means to be human.

One reading of Tournier's approach in this respect is that it is theologically naïve, a conviction of the usefulness of the Bible based largely on his own experience of the effectiveness of both individual and group

Bible study. Certainly, as just noted, he made no attempt to meet the challenges either of radical biblical criticism or of the extensive theological questioning of his time. Consistently with the degree of self-revelation required of the doctor in medicine of the person, Tournier frequently described in his writings his own beliefs and personal spiritual practice, but he always avoided theological controversy.

A different, and we believe more accurate, reading of Tournier's approach, is simply that it is strongly practical rather than theoretical in focus. Tournier was concerned not with the niceties of theological argument but with helping real people in real difficulties in the real world. This practical focus comes through particularly clearly in his attitude to beliefs and faiths that were different from his own. Although for his own part deeply influenced by his specifically Christian faith, he was at the same time fully open to the richness and diversity of other cultures and other faith traditions. He was aware for example that non-believers may show 'greater respect and understanding for the spiritual life of their patients than do some religious fanatics' (Tournier 1973, p.4).

Tournier, then, combined in medicine of the person a deep personal Christian conviction with a full and respectful openness to other beliefs and faith traditions. In this he was no doubt much influenced by his wide travels and equally wide reading. But as Robert Atwell, a Parish priest in London, and Bill Fulford show in their chapter 'The Christian Tradition of Spiritual Direction as a Sketch for a Strong Theology of Diversity', as the opening chapter (Chapter 6) of Part 2, this same openness, far from being antithetical to Christian conviction, is a central feature of a Christian tradition of spiritual direction, focused like medicine of the person on the practical needs of people of any faith or of no faith at all, stretching right back to the Desert Fathers of the early Christian church. The tradition of spiritual direction, indeed, as Atwell and Fulford illustrate in an extended case study that runs through their chapter, offers a rich resource of theory and practice for responding effectively to people's spiritual needs in contemporary pastoral and clinical care.

There is, though, considerably more to medicine of the person being 'for all faiths' than mere compatibility. For as the remaining chapters of Part 2 of the book show in different ways, medicine of the person, although indeed grounded originally on Christianity, is positively and powerfully enriched by the insights of other faiths. Thus Claire Hilton and Michael Hilton (Chapter 7), respectively an old-age psychiatrist and a Rabbi, while noting that Tournier's writings cannot be directly translated into a Jewish context, argue that they can nonetheless be usefully interpreted through a Jewish perspective. Key insights from Judaism for medicine of the person include an emphasis on deeds more than faith, a recognition of the dangers of professionalism undermining community, and the example of the Rabbi, as a cultural as well as religious figure, being adopted as a full and valued member of the health care team. Community is the focus, too, of the Egyptian psychiatrist, Ahmed Okasha in his account of the importance of the family in Islamic and traditional societies (Chapter 8). Okasha thus broadens medicine of the person from Tournier's focus on the doctor–patient dyad to the essential setting of that dyad in the context of the family and the community, a context that, with our perhaps excessive emphasis on individual rights, is surely in much need of fuller acknowledgement as the basis of a more balanced approach to health care decision-making. More radical still is the British psychiatrist Dinesh Bhugra's account of Hindu concepts of the person (Chapter 9). These concepts, as developed within the only non-Mediterranean religion represented in the book, challenge the taken-for-granted unity of the person in Western thinking, and thus, as Bhugra shows, bring us back through a very different spiritual route to the need for wholeness that is at the heart of the healing process in medicine of the person.

Taken together, the four chapters of Part 2 draw out the contemporary relevance of medicine of the person in a further respect, namely that, with every advance in the biological sciences it becomes more, not less, important to focus equally strongly on the psychosocial and spiritual aspects of health care. This is partly a matter of their causal interconnectedness: Jewish medicine has always been highly pragmatic in this respect; and both Okasha and Bhugra note recent research in the new neurosciences that is beginning to define some of the specific biological pathways, notably in the brain, mediating social and psychological processes.

However, the importance of emphasizing the psychosocial and spiritual equally with the biological is also a matter of practical effectiveness. Good medical practice requires that attention is given to the person of the patient and to establishing a genuinely human relationship between patient and doctor. This involves considering all facets of the person, including their beliefs (faiths) and spiritual understandings. This insight, of the importance of the whole person, although at the heart of the Christian tradition of spiritual direction and the clear message of other faith traditions, has still to be re-learned not only in 'Western' medicine but even, to some extent, in pastoral counselling. As noted earlier, pastoral counselling in the 1950s and 1960s followed other forms of counselling and psychotherapy at the time in developing 'non-directive' approaches. By the 1970s, pastoral counselling was beginning to grow out of its love affair with non-directiveness and to return to its roots in theology and biblical imagery (Campbell 1981). But even today, pastoral counselling remains a long way from re-establishing its place as a full faith-partner to the sciences in the healing process. Once again, time makes Tournier freshly relevant!

Relevance for contemporary medical practice

It is the relevance of medicine of the person for specific aspects of contemporary health care practice that is the focus of Part 3 of the book. As already noted, the contemporary relevance of medicine of the person is evident, not least, in the parallel between the central importance of the person in Tournier's work and the present-day demand for more person-centred care. Consistently with the inter-faith themes of Part 2, a recent study published in the *British Medical Journal* (Tarrant *et al.* 2003) and the subsequent correspondence (Unger, Ghilbert and Fisher 2003), has shown that a more person-centred approach is important across a wide range of cultures and faith traditions. The study in question, which was carried out in six general practices in Leicestershire representing diverse cultural and ethnic groups, used qualitative methods to explore patients' perceptions of personal care and whether or not a continuing relationship between health professional and patient was essential. The authors concluded that in all six practices human communication and person-centred approaches were important in making care genuinely personal, and that most respondents valued relationships in primary care and had clear ideas when care in the context of a relationship was most valuable.

Individualized person-centred care, then, is important across a wide range of different cultural contexts, including traditional family- or community-centred cultures as well as those that, as in Western Europe and North America, are strongly individual-centred (Okasha 2000). Again, Tournier, despite his focus on the doctor–patient dyad, anticipated the modern development of team working. In *A Listening Ear*, for example, Tournier, directly foreshadowing some of the policy developments in the UK's NHS noted earlier, refers to the possibility of a 'Hospital of the Person' (Tournier 1986, p.74).

Medicine of the person, however, is relevant not only in these broad brush ways to contemporary practice, important as person-centred care and team-working undoubtedly are, but also to a number of the unique and particular features of modern health care systems. It is with a sample of these unique and particular features that the five chapters making up Part 3 of the book are concerned. Spirituality in health care is, appropriately with the focus of Tournier's work, the first of these. Peter Gilbert (Chapter 10), a former social services director and now the national lead on spirituality for the National Institute for Mental Health in England (NIMHE) (the part of the UK's NHS responsible for delivering on policy in mental health), describes recent initiatives supported by central government policies for bringing the resources of the faith traditions more directly into health and social care.

Gilbert focuses on developments particularly in mental health: in England and Wales, for example, 'mindedness', based on meditative practices derived from Eastern religions, is proving a powerful ally of cognitive-behavioural approaches. This is consistent with Bhugra's observation in Chapter 9 that 'mindedness' and other techniques of meditation are proving helpful to many as part of a whole person approach to recovery in mental health. But in Scotland, which is subject to a different Health Executive, provision for patients' spiritual needs in all areas of health care has been put on a statutory (i.e. legally mandatory) basis (NHS Scotland, 2002). Similarly, within primary care, Tournier's own discipline, the Swiss family doctor Thierry Collaud (Chapter 11) shows how theological sources support the need for modern family medicine to move beyond the traditional doctor–patient dyad, which as we have noted was at the heart of all European medicine in Tournier's day, into the more complex context provided by the family and wider community.

Tom Fryers, an experienced British public health physician, shows the importance of spirituality even, and not least, in the health-economics dominated disciplines of public health (Chapter 12). Mike Magee, writing from a US perspective about health care particularly in older people, shows how technology, directly reflecting Tournier's marriage of science and faith, far from dehumanizing medicine is an increasingly powerful ally in providing person-centred primary care (Chapter 13). And the British psychiatrist Andrew Sims brings us back, finally, to the irreducible importance of the spiritual aspects of health care in scientific medicine, with his exploration of the issues raised by the challenge of reconciling a genuinely person-centred approach with the remarkable advances in behavioural genetics, personality-altering drugs and functional brain imaging that make up the new neurosciences (Chapter 14).

Conclusions

We have outlined in this introductory chapter how Tournier's work, although produced in the middle decades of the twentieth century, at a time when faith and science had become alienated in medicine, is increasingly relevant today. It is a mark of the richness of Tournier's thinking that, as the chapters in Part 1 of the book indicate, his work is relevant today not only in its own right but also as a living tradition that is sustained through the work of the International Medicine of the Person Group in Europe and the US, as well as the Paul Tournier Association based in Geneva. It is a mark of the richness of Tournier's thinking, in addition, that as the chapters in Part 2 illustrate, his work is relevant today not just in the predominantly Christian context in which he worked but also within the diverse and multi-faith context of contemporary practice. And it is a mark of the richness of Tournier's thinking, finally, that as the chapters in Part 3 indicate, his work is relevant today not just to our understanding of the relationship between doctors and their patients, the predominant mode of service delivery in Tournier's time, but also to our understanding of the far more complex services – multi-disciplinary, public health oriented, technologically supported, and the like – that are the basis of modern health care practice.

Sims' concluding chapter, though, in bringing us back at the end of the book to what we called earlier the twin pillars of medicine of the person, faith and science, points to what is perhaps the most enduring, and certainly the most vital, lesson of Tournier's work for contemporary health care, namely that, as resources for healing, faith and science, contrary to their alienation through much of the twentieth-century, and notwithstanding the intellectual challenges they continue to pose for philosophy, for theology and for the empirical sciences, are nonetheless fully reconciled in the relationships between the real people; the people who use services and the people who provide them, the real people who are at the heart of healing.

References

Beauchamp, T. and Childress, J. (1994) *Principles of Biomedical Ethics*, 4th edn. Oxford: Oxford University Press.

Bhugra, D. (ed) (1996) *Psychiatry and Religion*. London: Routledge.

Bonhoeffer, D. (1959) *Letters and Papers from Prison*. London: Fontana.

Brown, M.M., Brown, G.C. and Sharma, S. (2005) *Evidence-Based to Value-Based Medicine*. Chicago: American Medical Association Press.

Campbell, A.V. (1975) *Moral Dilemmas in Medicine*. London: Churchill.

Campbell, A.V. (1981) *Rediscovering Pastoral Care*. London: Darton, Longman & Todd.

Cox, J.L. (1996) 'Psychiatry and Religion: A General Psychiatrist's Perspective.' In D. Bhugra (ed) *Psychiatry and Religion*. London: Routledge.

Culliford, L. (2002) 'Spiritual care and psychiatric treatment: an introduction.' *Advances in Psychiatric Treatment 18*, 249–263.

Department of Health (2003a) *Inspiring Hope: Recognising the Importance of Spirituality in a Whole Person Approach to Mental Health*. National Institute for Mental Health in England. Web: www.nimhe.org.uk.

Department of Health (2003b) *Meeting the Spiritual and Religious Needs of Patients and Staff: Guidance for Staff*. London: HMSO.

Department of Health (2004) (40339) *The Ten Essential Shared Capabilities: A Framework for the Whole of the Mental Health Workforce*. London: The Sainsbury Centre for Mental Health, the NHSU (National Health Service University) and the NIMHE (National Institute for Mental Health England).

Department of Health (2005) *Creating a Patient-led NHS: Delivering the NHS Improvement Plan*. London: Department of Health.

Dickenson, D. and Fulford, K.W.M. (2000) *In Two Minds: A Casebook of Psychiatric Ethics*. Oxford: Oxford University Press.

Editorial (2004) 'The soft science of medicine.' *Lancet 363*, 1247.

Fulford, K.W.M (1996) 'Religion and Psychiatry: Extending the Limits of Tolerance'. In D. Bhugra (ed) *Psychiatry and Religion*. London: Routledge.

Fulford, K.W.M. (2004) 'Ten principles of values-based medicine.' In J. Radden (ed) *The Philosophy of Psychiatry: A Companion*. New York: Oxford University Press.

Fulford, K.W.M., Thornton, T. and Graham, G. (2006) 'From bioethics to values-based practice'. In K.W.M. Fulford, T. Thornton and G. Graham *The Oxford Textbook of Philosophy and Psychiatry*. Oxford: Oxford University Press.

Haering, B. (1972) *Medical Ethics*. Slough: St Paul Press.

Hunink, M., Glasziou, P., Siegel, J., Weeks, J., Pliskin, J., Elstein, A. and Weinstein, M. (2001) *Decision Making in Health and Medicine: Integrating Evidence and Values*. Cambridge: Cambridge University Press.

McCormick, R. (1981) *How Brave a New World?* London: SCM Press.

National Framework of Values for Mental Health (not dated) National Institute for Mental Health in England. Available at: kc.nimhe.org.uk/upload/NIMHE%20Values%20Framework.pdf.

NHS Scotland (2002) *Spiritual Care in the NHS Scotland.* Edinburgh: NHS Scotland. [ref HDL (2002) 76].

Okasha, A. (2000) 'The Impact of Arab Culture on Psychiatric Ethics.' In A. Okasha, J. Arboleda-Florez and N. Sartorius (eds) *Ethics, Culture and Psychiatry.* Washington: American Psychiatric Press.

Ramsey, P. (1970) *The Patient as a Person.* London: Yale University Press.

Rogers, C. (1961) *On Becoming a Person.* New York: Houghton Mifflin.

Singer, P. (1993) *Practical Ethics.* Cambridge: Cambridge University Press.

Tarrant, C., Windridge, K., Boulton, M., Baker, R. and Freeman, G. (2003) 'Qualitative study of the meaning of personal care in General Practice.' *British Medical Journal, 326,* 1310.

Tillich, P. (1953) *Systematic Theology,* Vol. I. London: Nisbet.

Tournier, P. (1954) *A Doctor's Casebook in the Light of the Bible.* London: SCM Press.

Tournier, P. (1957) *The Meaning of Persons.* London: SCM Press.

Tournier, P. (1957 [1940]) *Médicine de la Personne.* Neuchâtel and Paris: Delachaux et Niestlé.

Tournier, P. (1962) *Guilt and Grace.* London: Hodder and Stoughton.

Tournier, P. (1973) 'The doctor, the senior citizen and the meaning of life.' *Journal of Psychology and Theology 1,* 4–9.

Tournier, P. (1986) *A Listening Ear: Fifty Years as a Doctor of the Whole Person.* Texts selected by Charles Piguet. London: Hodder and Stoughton.

Unger, J.P., Ghilbert, P. and Fisher, J.P. (2003) 'Doctor–patient communication in developing countries: do what I do, not what I say.' *British Medical Journal 327,* 450.

Woodbridge, K. and Fulford, K.W.M. (2003) 'Good practice? Values-based practice in mental health.' *Mental Health Practice 7,* 2, 30–34.

PART I

MEDICINE OF THE PERSON: PAUL TOURNIER'S VISION

CHAPTER 2

THE MAN AND HIS MESSAGE

Hans-Rudolf Pfeifer and John Cox

Introduction

Paul Tournier (1898–1986), physician and writer from Geneva, Switzerland, made an outstanding pioneering contribution to the understanding and practice of an integrative approach of medicine, psychology and pastoral counselling, which had an impact on many professionals and laymen alike in all continents. He was the founder of 'Médecine de la Personne' ('Medicine of the Person').

His work and the message of medicine of the person is best understood against the background of his biography. His attitude and challenge were derived from his own experiences, yet we believe are equally valid for health care systems across the world that are striving to meet the wish of patients and service users for more person-centred and holistic health care.

Family upbringing

Paul Tournier was born on 12 May 1898. His father Louis Tournier died only two months later at the age of 70. He had been a much appreciated Calvinistic pastor in the Cathedral of Saint Peter in Geneva. Paul Tournier's mother Elizabeth, born Ormond, was Louis' much younger second wife. Unfortunately she died at the age of 42 from breast cancer, thus leaving Paul an orphan at six. He described the loss of his mother as without doubt 'the most important event of my childhood' (Tournier 1986, p.127); 'When my mother died I felt like vanishing in a black hole of nothingness' (Tournier 1982b). He felt painful emptiness and was afraid of being totally insignificant to anybody in the future.

He thus lost the loving, intellectual and religious influence of his first home, and together with his 10-year-old sister was moved into the environment of the worldly business family of his uncle and aunt, Mr and Mrs Jacques Ormond, who had previously lost two children of their own. Paul was unable to accept affection, he withdrew into himself. He was very lonely. He felt he did not count as a person and that no one liked him. At school he was ridiculed by his classmates. Except for mathematics he was a poor student. At the same time he was very practically minded and talented in all manual things. His uncle advised him to learn something practical and not to study later on. He had no friends, instead he preferred playing with his uncle's dog and to retreat in his own tree house. In his own eyes he was 'a disturbed child' quite likely to develop mental health problems. He suffered from his loneliness and felt he did not really exist ('Je n'existais pas') (Tournier 1986, p.128). Furthermore his aunt whom he grew up with was affected with intermittent severe mental disorders.

When he was 12 years of age he decided for himself to become a medical doctor. As Tournier recognized later, his mind saw medicine as a career through which he could overcome his loneliness and find contact with people. Perhaps this was an unconscious decision to fight the sickness and death which had taken his mother from him (Tournier 1986). He also took a decision to commit his life more consciously to God. 'I wanted to find my own identity and I wanted to find a father in God, having missed my father so much on this earth' (Tournier 1982b).

A key experience happened at the age of 16. His Greek teacher Jules Dubois invited him home for a visit. He took time to talk with him, to listen to him and gave him the opportunity to open up and to discover himself more. 'He introduced me to dialogue and saved me from my loneliness' (Tournier 1986, p.131). Paul felt like never before, his teacher took him seriously and respected his ideas. 'He gave me the feeling that I existed' ('Il m'a fait exister!') (Tournier 1982b). Paul was invited back almost every week for nearly ten years. For Paul this continuous dialogue was like a first level of becoming a person. It was an intellectual dialogue, an exchange of thoughts and ideas. They did not talk about personal things from their private lives. Only later did he understand that his teacher had been like a psychotherapist to him.

The transformation that took place was evident. It gave him enough self-confidence to move more into society. He started to participate passionately in public discussions, for example on intellectual and political issues. It was the time of the First World War and of the Russian Revolution. He participated in a theatre group of his school, performing in Greek, Latin and French. He wrote and performed a play on the Swiss apostle of peace Niklaus von der Flüe. He also got involved in social activities.

Medical studies

From 1917 to 1923 he studied medicine at the University of Geneva. He not only stood out as a leading figure of the student movement in Geneva but became the Swiss president of the Zofingia Student Association, which celebrated its centenary in 1920/1921. In this function he enjoyed giving public speeches in different cities of Switzerland. Furthermore he served with the Red Cross in Vienna for the repatriation of Russian, Austrian and German prisoners of war. He organized fund-raising for child welfare work in famine-stricken Russia. He was co-founder of a home for mothers with their children, suffering from tuberculosis.

Looking back on this period of his life, he stated:

> I had found a relationship with society, but on an intellectual level. However I was still hiding my inner loneliness. I could lead discussions in front of thousands of people, but I was unable to enter into a deeper personal relationship. (Tournier 1982b)

After completing his medical studies he was an intern in Paris and in Geneva. He opened his own private general practice in 1925.

Marriage to Nelly

In 1924 he married Nelly Bouvier in Geneva. They had known each other for many years. She was maybe less trained intellectually and she certainly expressed a lot of admiration for Paul. She reflected on their early relationship as follows: 'You are my teacher, my doctor, my psychologist, my pastor, but you are not my husband' (Tournier 1986, p.132). Paul commented:

> She was not talking about our intimate relationship, which was fine. Rather she meant by that, that I was too intellectual, holding talks, giving private lectures to her. I presented a lot of knowledge in science, psychology, and theology, but I could not develop true fellowship with her. My escape into intellectualism was my problem. I had found my way on an intellectual basis, but the personal, the

affective emotional dimension was still hidden and closed to me.
(Tournier 1982b)

This was going to change a lot later on.

Two sons were born: Jean-Louis in 1925 and Gabriel in 1928. Jean
Louis stayed single and worked for the Post Office. Over the years he was
very much involved as a volunteer for the Olympic office and museum in
Lausanne. He died in 2001. Gabriel became an architect and built the
'Grain de Blé' (Corn of Wheat), as Paul Tournier's house in Troinex near
Geneva was called. His wife Monique was a painter-artist and died in
2003. They have four children and several grandchildren. Gabriel and his
son Alain are co-founders and members of the Paul Tournier Association
since 1998, with the aim of collecting books, tapes, films, pictures and
further written materials related to Paul Tournier, making them accessible
to research and intending to further his views and impact in present
times.

Church work and the Oxford Group

Paul Tournier also became very involved in the church. He was active in a
group of laymen and clergy who were discussing ways to revitalize the
church. He was elected to the church governing body where he got into
fiery debates struggling for the right interpretation of faith and a return to
basic reformed Christianity. But all his well-meant efforts did not seem to
lead to any good, it rather caused struggle and divisions. He finally withdrew from his involvement in the church government and had an increasing feeling of needing a change in his life.

In 1932 Paul Tournier had an encounter that would transform him,
with long-lasting effects. He was treating a very difficult patient with
psychological problems who quite unexpectedly changed for the better.
Almost overnight her egotism and aggressive manner had given way to
kindness and devotion to others. She told him that she had participated in
a seminar organized by a new religiously oriented movement from Oxford; this helped her to deeper personal insights and to personal change.
Dr Tournier asked his patient to introduce him to representatives of that
movement. In Geneva on 24 November 1932 he met with Emil Brunner,
Professor of Theology; Alfons Maeder, Psychoanalyst; Theophil Spörri,
Professor of Literature – all renowned people in their fields from Zürich –

and Jan de Bordes, a finance expert in the League of Nations (Tournier 1986).

The Oxford Movement had started among students from Oxford. The founder was Frank Buchmann who underlined the importance of religious faith put into practice in personal and public life, rather than stressing dogmas and theories. People were encouraged to meditate for a period of time each day and to seek inner guidance in practical details of life. In small groups people would exchange personal experiences, trying to develop more openness, honesty and transparency.

That remarkable night Tournier had expected an intellectual discussion on the principles of the movement and to learn more about the secrets of its success. Instead these men were silent for half an hour, followed by a very personal time of sharing experiences as well as failures in their own lives. Tournier was disappointed at first, however he was also deeply touched by this way of sharing with each other.

Shortly after that he met again with Jan de Bordes who shared with him very personally about his life. When he finished, Tournier realized he could not just talk about his activities, rather he had to talk really about himself, about his own personal life:

> For the first time in my life and under tears I talked about my inner suffering as an orphan. For the first time in 34 years I cried over my mother, I cried over my father. It was the second level of becoming more of a person, not just the intellectual reflection of ideas, but rather the emotional encounter from person to person. (Tournier 1982b)

He discovered a different way of dialogue integrating the emotional side. It was a liberating experience for him, talking about himself, not just about opinions in books and intellectual knowledge but rather about existential experience.

Tournier discovered in the approach of the Oxford Movement parallels to the psychotherapeutic process. 'I opened up to friends about my life, my feelings, my fears, about my shames and my longings. Without being conscious of it, there was everything that constitutes psychotherapy: catharsis, emotional discharge, awareness and transference' (Tournier 1982a, pp.35–36). Beyond that it also included very personal religious experiences, characterized by a closeness to 'the love and grace of God' like he had not known it before.

Meditation

From then on Paul Tournier spent one hour per day in silence. He would write down some notes if some thoughts and impressions crossed his mind. To him it was the beginning of a lifelong journey of inner listening that would balance and redirect his outward activities. It was 'an attitude of openness, a willingness to listen to God' (Tournier 1986, p.12ff). He also meditated on texts, especially biblical texts, but not in a systematic way. He always tried to put the results of his quiet time, of his inner collection, as small as they may have been, into practice in his life. His wife also started sharing in this, each one for themselves and occasionally together.

General practice and psychotherapy

This daily discipline transformed his marriage and family, his relationships to others and also to his patients. It changed his private practice. Without him telling the patients what had happened to him, they started opening up to him in a way they never did before.

> I believe people have an intuitive ability: they share with us what we are ready to receive. When I approached them intellectually, they only brought up intellectual questions. But if you have walked a deeper process in your soul, they open up and share their deeper problems which they have been hiding thus far. ('Ils nous apportent ce que l'on est prêt a recevoir', Tournier 1982b)

He felt he needed more time for his patients and invited some back in the evenings, talking with them by his fireplace, something for which Tournier became very famous. During a few years he lived a 'daylife' where he treated his patients as a doctor and an 'evening life' where he encountered his patients in a deeper sense person to person. He tried to integrate the aspects of science and faith, of medical doctor and counsellor.

He became curious about investigating further how a personal relationship between doctor and patient could contribute to his or her health and what the significance of personal religious experience could be for medical practice. In 1937 he wrote a letter to all of his patients informing them about the new focus of his private practice. Quite a few patients changed to another general practitioner, but at the same time many doctors would send him their most difficult psychosomatic cases.

He never had formal training in the psychiatric field or in a particular psychotherapeutic school. As much as he had become interested and specialized in that domain, he deepened his knowledge and experience through books and friends very much in an autodidactic way. He did ask well-known Alphonse Maeder and Theo Bovet, both psychoanalysts who had been in direct touch with Sigmund Freud and Carl Gustav Jung, whether he should undertake training in psychoanalysis. Both gave him the same answer, realizing his great counselling potential: 'We are not short of good psychoanalysts, there are plenty of them; but we have only one Paul Tournier' (Tournier 1982a, pp.35–36).

They encouraged him to continue in his particular personal calling to pursue 'a synthesis of psychology, classical medicine and even religious belief'. To achieve such a synthesis he should not be bound to any particular doctrinal bias or prejudice, as in their view could be the case in formal psychoanalytic training. 'So there, I did not become a psychoanalyst; I opted for the medicine of the whole person, the non-specialized attitude *par excellence*, which seeks to understand man as a whole' (Tournier 1982a, pp.35–36).

Tournier as author

It was in 1940 that he published his first book under the French title which would become programmatic for his life: *Médecine de la Personne*. The German edition followed 1941, titled *Krankheit und Lebensprobleme* (illness and life problems); the English translation did not appear until quite a few years later: *The Healing of Persons* (1965). He had already written the first draft before the outbreak of World War II. He was called to service as a military doctor but continued to elaborate on his manuscript. Still very hesitant whether he should publish it, he was greatly encouraged by his friends to do so. He was surprised about the positive reactions. Further books followed, touching on existential themes that were at the core of his heart: *Escape from Loneliness*, 1962 (*De la Solitude à la Communauté*, 1943), or *The Person Reborn*, 1966 (*Technique et Foi*, 1946).

Little did he realize at first what positive echo his books would also find abroad. Only after the war had ended would he receive most encouraging letters, especially from Germany and Holland. In 1946 he experienced a painful separation from the Oxford Movement that had meant so much to his personal development. They had turned into 'Moral Rearmament', located in Caux near Vevey, Switzerland, and he realized that it had taken an ideological moralistic course that he could not identify with any more. He lost many friends with whom he had had close relationships before. (The movement has undergone significant further transitions, now called 'Initiatives of Change', contributing considerably to reconciliation processes in many parts of the world – see www.iofc.org). It was only in 1982 that Tournier went back to Caux and felt he could be reconciled with them.

In 1946 he and his wife were invited to Germany for a conference of medical doctors and counsellors in Bad Boll. He met with significant people such as Victor von Weizsäcker. In 1947 Tournier himself for the first time invited medical doctors to a one-week retreat at the ecumenical Institute Bossey near Geneva, for what he then called a 'Group for the Research on Medicine of the Person' ('Groupe de la Recherche de la Médecine de la Personne'). Conferences have since then taken place almost annually in different places in Europe. In 1969 the Group published an account of the first 20 years, which also included their summary of the core concepts of medicine of the person (Le Groupe Bossey 1969). The 57th meeting took place in Great Britain in 2005 and the 58th meeting took place in Switzerland in 2006. Other regular meetings are being held in the USA.

The participants have come from various professional backgrounds and *Weltanschauung* (views of life), although medical doctors of Christian background have been a majority. Tournier did not just want lectures and intellectual discussion, but he wanted to give opportunities for personal encounters and sharing, so people would not just discuss patients and opinions but open up about their personal questions and doubts, failures and joys. Tournier conducted a Bible study every morning of these conferences for many years, not as a theological exegesis, but as 'existential explication', which in their liveliness, practical approach and very personal dimension were unforgettable for those who had attended. In general, theologians were discouraged from attending, because Paul Tournier had noticed that doctors then talked less about their difficulties, spiritual experiences and clinical dilemmas. Other family members were however regarded as major influences on the person and practice of the doctor and were always welcomed. There were no accompanying persons at these gatherings, nor any simultaneous translation. Then as now the personalized translations into French, German and English are a core expressive experience of a meeting of the international Medicine of the Person Group.

Paul Tournier published further books (a total of 20), which have been translated into over 20 languages, sold millions of copies and have found a worldwide readership. He also wrote articles and gave radio interviews. All his books touched on existential themes such as *The Whole Person in a Broken World, The Strong and the Weak, A Doctor's Casebook in the Light of the Bible, The Meaning of Persons, To Resist or to Surrender*, etc. In his book *Guilt and Grace* (1962) he also refers to the tragic car accident when his uncle who brought him up was killed, while Paul Tournier was driving the car, in 1935. Towards his eighties he wrote books such as *Learning to Grow Old, The Gift of Feeling* (*La Mission de la Femme*) and *Creative Suffering*.

Overseas travel, ecumenism and interfaith issues

He was invited for speaking tours throughout the whole of Europe, to the USA, South Africa, but also to Japan and Muslim countries. His book *A Doctor's Casebook in the Light of the Bible* (1954) was approved by the Vatican and he was active in the early days of the Ecumenical movement in Switzerland.

Always he stood firm for his Christian roots, but was very tolerant and open to dialogue with anyone: atheists, Buddhists or Muslims alike. In Isfahan, Iran, he was even invited to talk in a Mosque. He observed that doctors could create a bond which transcended 'denominational boundaries, and even barriers between different religions'. Tournier recognized the possibility of uniting not only Christians but also Jews and Muslims in a 'spiritual view of man' (Tournier 1986, p.81).

He was offered professorships in USA and Geneva but turned them down every time. In his view 'Médecine de la Personne' could not really be taught from the pulpit, but rather be shared by personal example and experience. He was not in the contemporary sense an educationalist or researcher. Primarily he was an author and clinician; all life long he continued his private psychotherapeutic practice as a general practitioner. Many people gave testimony to the great help they had received, being led into more inner listening and responsibility of their own to deal with their own life's problems. He treated people from all walks of life, even one future President of the USA.

Death of Nelly and Paul Tournier

The death of his wife in 1974 during a conference in Athens was a great loss to him. 'It felt like I had become an orphan for the third time' (Tournier 1982b). She had meant so much to him in terms of his becoming more of a person and in terms of his learning to dialogue in deeper ways, as well as supporting his ministry.

He remained active and vital until old age. In 1984 he was remarried to a 50-year-old pianist, Corinne O'Rama from Geneva. Paul Tournier died on 7 October 1986 at his home in Troinex near Geneva, Switzerland, from a carcinoma, shortly after participating in a conference in Strasbourg.

Many people, especially in the medical, psychotherapeutic and psychiatric field, have testified to the impact Paul Tournier, through his books, speeches and the conferences on 'Medicine of the Person', has had on them. He had a vast correspondence and would answer each letter in a very personal way within a few days.

The basic attitudes and concepts of 'Médecine de la Personne' are relevant, and even more significant for contemporary health care, with its ethical dilemmas and tremendous technological advances, yet limited resources and dehumanizing dangers.

Viktor Frankl, the famous Viennese Psychiatrist and founder of Logotherapy and Existential Analysis, referred to Paul Tournier, saying:

> He was the pioneer of person-centred psychotherapy. Psychotherapy should also have a spiritual dimension, dealing with each person in his or her uniqueness and individuality. Psychotherapy cannot be personal enough; this is what Paul Tournier programmatically expressed in the title of his book *Médecine de la Personne*. (Frankl 1984, p.100)

Medicine of the person

For Tournier and his colleagues, 'Medicine of the Person' was an approach to medical care that emphasized attention being given to the whole person – to the biological, psychological, social *and* spiritual aspects of health problems. Good medical practice required that attention is given to the person of the patient, and to establishing a real relationship that considered all facets of the patient, including their beliefs (faiths) and spiritual understandings. In a phrase used by Juan Mezzich (2005), President of the World Psychiatric Associaton (WPA), it should be a 'Medicine of the Person, for the Person, by the Person, and with the Person'.

Tournier emphasized that developing spiritual sensitivity in the doctor was an essential component of medicine of the person. The international meetings were an opportunity where this growth could occur. He recognized that limited and timely self-disclosure may personalize a consultation in a way that was beneficial. The doctor–patient relationship was regarded by these Swiss doctors as spiritual in the sense expressed by Martin Buber who contrasted the 'I–Thou' relationship, which had a spiritual dimension, with the more impersonal 'I–It' encounter (Tournier 1978).

Tournier had an anecdotal, intimate and often personalized style of writing, as shown in the following extract from *The Meaning of Persons*:

> Even if I could arrive at a knowledge of all the physical, chemical, and biological phenomena of the body, all the psychical phenomena of the mind, and all the spiritual, social, historical and philosophical factors at work in man, would it make me into a doctor of the person? Would it result in personal contact with my patient? In the end of the day, I would still be in the world of things. Knowledge of things, even of an infinity of things, does not bring us to knowledge of the person... Do not misunderstand me; I am not denying the usefulness or the interest of the effort to synthesize our scientific knowledge of man. But, however successful, it will reveal only one side of man's nature: that of his mechanisms. It will still be necessary to complete it with a personal knowledge, which is of a different order, the order of the person, not that of things.
>
> This knowledge is within the reach of every doctor, be he an ordinary general practitioner or a learned specialist. (Tournier 1957, p.187)

The man and the message

Paul Tournier was aware of the risks of a mechanical reductionist medical practice, devoid of ethics and without sustaining compassion. The risks of such practice were plainly visible in post-war Europe. A reductionist approach to medicine restricted to biomedicine alone was, Tournier believed, not only dangerous but lacked the integration of body, mind and spirit necessary for health and wholeness. It also overlooked the healing that occurs in a therapeutic relationship. He anticipated the present-day search for a healing relationship in health care provision, and the recognition that spirituality cannot be neglected in the training of all health workers.

Medicine of the person was not a specialist technique confined to primary care, nor was it psychosomatic medicine or a school of counselling, but rather a personalized approach to patients and staff in a therapeutic team (Tournier 1968).

It is, we believe, an integrative, person-centered medicine that considers psychospiritual as well as biosocial aspects of patient care, and in particular recognizes the healing potential of a caring relationship.

Objectives of a medicine of the whole person are, among others:

> to help patients find the meaning of their sickness and their life; to deal with the problem of death; to discover a specific ethical approach to their environment; to open sources of love for themselves and for their fellow-men; to sense the meaning of suffering…to find strength through the community for a new responsibility towards themselves and their fellow-men. (Harnik 1973, p.14)

In *A Place for You* Tournier described medicine of the person as considering man in his relationship with the environment. Man was to be seen in relation and interaction with others, with the world and with God.

> Society, the world and God are his external place; his body, mind and spirit are his internal place. God has created us in our totality; he has given us our place; he rules over our physical as well as our spiritual lives…that is why among the followers of the Medicine of the Person there are not only psychiatrists and psychotherapists of every school of psychological medicine but also a great number of surgeons, and other specialists in physical medicine – ear, nose and throat specialists, ophthalmic surgeons, gastro-enterologists, and radiologists. (Tournier 1968, p.68)

Interestingly, Ben Harnik broadened further the ideas of Tournier by suggesting that this way of approaching others may also be relevant for other professions such as teachers, lawyers and social workers (1973, p.14).

Yet as we have described in this chapter, the development and the relevance of medicine of the person cannot be separated from an understanding of Dr Paul Tournier the man. Indeed the man was also the message – and the message was also in the man.

References

Frankl, V.E. (1984) *Der leidende Mensch. Anthropologische Grundlagen der Psychotherapie.* Bern Stuttgart Toronto: Verlag Hans Huber.

Harnik, B. (ed) (1973) *Paul Tournier's Medicine of the Whole Person. 39 Essays.* Waco, Texas: Word Books.

Le Groupe de Bossey (1969) *Vingt Annees de Medecine de la Personne.* Chantec: Melun D.

Mezzich, J.E. (2005) *Science and Humanism; A Double Helix for the Future of Psychiatry.* Plenary Lecture, XIII World Congress of Psychiatry, Cairo.

Tournier, P. (1954) *A Doctor's Casebook in the Light of the Bible.* London: SCM Press.

Tournier, P. (1957) *The Meaning of Persons: Reflections on a Psychiatrist's Casebook.* London: SCM Press.

Tournier, P. (1968) *A Place for You.* London: SCM Press.

Tournier, P. (1978) 'Relationships: The third dimension of medicine.' In Christian Medical Commission, *Contact Bulletin 47*, Geneva: World Council of Churches.

Tournier, P. (1982a) *Creative Suffering.* London: SCM Press.

Tournier, P. (1982b) *Médecine de la Personne – My Personal Way as Christian and as a Doctor.* Lecture held in Zurich, Switzerland on 12 May. Tape at Paul Tournier Association, CH-1256 Troinex/Geneva.

Tournier, P. (1986) *A Listening Ear: Fifty Years as a Doctor of the Whole Person.* Texts selected by Charles Piguet.

CHAPTER 3

RETAINING THE PERSON IN MEDICAL SCIENCE

Bernard Rüedi

Introduction

Never has medicine appeared as efficient as it does today, and its recent technical performances anticipate even more impressive applications for the future. Proud of its successes, does our current medical practice still keep the suffering person as its main concern and meet all his or her needs?

Of course, we must agree that it is now often claimed that medicine has to be patient-centred, and the terms of personalized or individualized medicine appear more and more frequently in the scientific literature. However, if patient-centred health care has to be individualized, this does not mean that it is also person-centred. Individualized care takes into account treatments adjusted to the various characteristics of the sick patient, mainly his or her inherited and acquired biological specificities. These are qualities proper to a sick individual; they have to be cured – but the person has also to be met, helped and healed.

Indeed, the image of a healing person has always been evoked in the mind of the suffering person. Its archetype is shaped into different representations: priest, sorcerer, shaman, medicine man and doctor, according to the various cultural backgrounds of the populations. Since the physician is supposed to be able to save the patient from death, he also obtains in the process some qualities of a divine and omnipotent entity.

Of course, today everyone knows that this representation is irrational, but the unconscious expectations of the patient still keep this hope in mind; medical science has to become more and more efficient, to allow people to live longer and better, even with partly artificial bodies, as if life expectancy is the main human value. We say we know that the risk of dying is 100 per cent but we behave as if we had forgotten it, arguing that we are conscious to talk only about a risk of premature death.

On the other hand, we must also agree that sometimes the physician also takes advantage of the powerful image projected onto him and does little to prevent or to correct it.

Finally, the sometimes understandable but frequently excessive rejection of an efficient scientific medicine and the interest in alternative medicines may also express the objection of the patient to being only an object of care. If the suffering patient is today strongly asking for the best technical treatment, he or she is also hoping that it would be provided through a personal physician–patient relationship.

Since the patient of today is expecting both an efficient treatment and to be recognized and met as a suffering person, our present medicine must succeed in answering both requests; neither can be excluded. Both have to be efficient and complementary. If the physician of today wants to keep enough time to meet the person of his patient and master the growing scientific knowledge needed in his daily practice, he will not be able to memorize more and more information but will have to learn new methods to access the right knowledge when needed.

Paul Tournier and Medicine of the Person

In 1940, Paul Tournier, a general practitioner, published a book, *Médecine de la Personne*, and soon after founded a group bearing the same name. At that time medical science looked already very promising, but psychosomatics was only at its very beginning. Sixty years later, the former has kept its promises and the latter has won acclaim. However, personalized medicine, bearing in mind all the facets of the patient, and psychosomatics cannot and must not replace medicine of the person, which favours a more specific approach to the patient.

Martin Buber (1960) distinguishes the 'I–It' me from the 'I–Thou' me. The first one, with his or her ever-incomplete knowledge of the world and of his or her own person, which is mainly unconscious, tries to describe and apprehend the things and the people. The second one, on the contrary, discovers with his or her whole person the whole person of the other. With his 'I–It' me, man can and must take possession of the world he has been placed in. But in the dialogue the 'I–Thou' man will discover the true expectations of the other: his or her fears, the meaning he or she is giving to their own life – in other words, the richness of the other – and become even enriched by it. The specificity of medicine of the person is to integrate this dimension and, according to the true biological effect that the prescription of a placebo can induce, such an empathic approach may well be characterized as a 'therapeutic relationship'.

Beside conventional medical consultations in his office, Paul Tournier sometimes gave to his patients an opportunity of 'discussion in the chimney-corner', allowing more personal dialogues where the label of the physician was left behind. These conversations did not follow the rules of psychotherapeutic or psychoanalytic procedures, but they permitted both persons to really make acquaintance. The patient was feeling that he was understood and loved, and the doctor could better understand the impact and the meaning of the disease for his patient.

Of course, such an approach induced a psychotherapeutic relationship and some psychiatrists have reproached Paul Tournier for having performed psychotherapy without having being trained for it, but fortunately others dissuaded him from undergoing personal psychoanalysis or specific training in psychotherapy, arguing the fact that he would no longer be Paul Tournier.

Paul Tournier included very often a spiritual dimension when meeting the patient, but this does not mean that all physicians should behave like him. Paul Tournier was neither a psychiatrist, nor a 'conventional' general practitioner. He was Paul Tournier, practising a specific kind of medical relationship, which cannot be copied, but his example encourages us to take into account a specific and decisive dimension to integrate into the therapeutic relationship.

Indeed, Paul Tournier believed that man couldn't avoid the spiritual questions about his own life, sickness and death. To practise medicine of the person and meet the suffering person with his or her essential preoccupations, it is necessary to be prepared to share also the spiritual ones. That requires having, if possible, a strong personal spiritual reference to lean upon, and without being exclusive, the Christian reference remains the most natural and immediate in our Western culture. Paul Tournier practised meditation every morning with his wife, sharing with her their complementary ways of feeling the words of God.

Paul Tournier had a Christ-centred view of medicine of the person but he always claimed that Christians were not the exclusive guardians of medicine of the person. He had also met true physicians of the person in other cultures who were also leaning upon a spiritual reference, for example in Buddhism, where compassion and love are central values.

Aloys von Orelli, a Swiss Jungian psychiatrist (1909–1997) and active participant in the group since the beginning, explained that, in our culture, it was in discovering and meeting the person of God that man could better understand the significance and the meaning of his acts and of his life, also having the possibility of better choices, even in his medical practice (Orelli 1974).

Man, said Aloys von Orelli, is destined to discover his whole person, in the image of God's person, and it begins to become possible after having experienced a personal meeting with Him. But man, fascinated by his 'I–It' power to master nature and life, drives the world towards destruction. The same fate could occur for the medicine if its only goal were to cure diseases. Unfortunately it is vain to imagine that society might collectively bring this knowledge into conscience. Only if more and more people, individually, become conscious of the meaning and the consequences of their acts and choices, will our society be allowed if not to prevent, at least to delay the disaster.

Our true responsibilities are individual, said Orelli, and everyone has to walk towards his whole person, by the discovery of God's person; in the meeting He offers us to be able later on to work in the world, following His example.

Paul Tournier, as a patient, was also able to meet the person of his doctor, promoting the reciprocity in the physician–patient dialogue, and I have had the privilege to discover it when he was hospitalized in my department.

To meet the person of the other requires meeting him or her where he or she is, and how he or she is, and not as we would like him or her to be. We must accept his or her total freedom to even refuse a 'true personal relationship', and in such a situation we can only be there and available.

This can be sometimes quite difficult and frustrating. I remember a young anorectic patient we had followed with a psychiatrist for several years, who had already made several attempts at suicide, and who told us: 'I agree to meet you again but only if you promise me that if I decide to commit suicide you will not force me to live.' We accepted. This happened several years ago, and the medical relationship is still continuing.

Practising medicine of the person does not allow, however, for leaving mastery of scientific knowledge and technologies to second position. On the contrary, it must bring the physician to offer his patient the best and 'individualized' therapeutic means, chosen and applied during a personalized meeting with him or her.

However, facing the tremendous increase and renewal of scientific knowledge, how will the physician manage to master it without sacrificing the time needed and an open mind for personal encounters?

Personalized medicine is not yet a medicine of the person

In 'Challenge of personal health care: to what extent is medicine already individualized and what are the future trends?', Walter Fierz (2004, p.111) says that 'the personal aspects of health care have been partly neglected in the current era of evidence-based scientific medicine. We now know that a "one fits all" type of treatment has its limits. Medicine needs to be re-personalized'. And he states further: 'The challenge is to regain individualism on a scientific base. Individualized medicine has to be based on evidence'.

In the case of an infectious disease, for example, Fierz suggests that personalized medicine can be conceptualized along several dimensions:

1. the disease

2. the environment

3   the genes, which means the molecular traits and mechanisms underlining the individual characteristics of both the patient and the microbe

4. the medication – pharmacogenomic studies will develop therapeutic agents targeted to specific, genetically identifiable subgroups of populations

5. the health care process including genetic counselling, the education of the patient and of his or her risk profile, a shared decision and the monitoring of the treatment, etc.

6. information management, both patient specific and evidence-based.

(Fierz 2004, p.112–115)

One can fully agree with such an approach to the sick patient, which needs to collect not only biological but also very personal information about the patient and his or her environment, and his or her social, professional and familial position. However, Paul Tournier required more than this. The dimensions mentioned above are essential for efficient treatment of the patient, but they concern only his disease. They do not reach his core.

Up until now the statements of evidence-based medicine have been established from the results of double-blind and randomized studies. These attempt to eliminate all subjective ideas and suggestions that might influence patients' or doctors' opinions. Either when comparing two drugs, or one drug against a placebo, the prescription of the medication has to be as 'neutral' as possible so that only the 'biological effect' becomes evident. The difference between what has happened with the drug and with the placebo is then considered as a true biological effect.

However, is it really true? The placebo effect is always considered as a wrong and unfounded impression of the subject, who is convinced that the expected effect has happened. Several observations have, however, clearly demonstrated that a placebo pill can induce a documented biological effect.

In 1978, Levine performed an interesting study: two groups of subjects about to have a dental extraction received either a placebo alone or a placebo combined with naloxone. The expected and observed analgesic effect of the placebo was negated by the addition of naloxone, showing that the placebo was able to release endorphins in the brain of the subjects. Other studies have also demonstrated the true biological effect of a placebo in Parkinson's disease and depression.

These observations show that what is called 'a therapeutic relationship' is not just compassion and a warm and attentive attitude, but that it may induce a true biological effect, either positive or negative. The attitude and the confidence in prescribing and receiving the prescription of a drug can amplify or neutralize its biological effect. These observations also draw attention to the careful interpretation of the results of the studies, since the placebo pill can also induce the expected biological effects.

Quoting these studies in his book *La Force de Guérir* (The strength for healing), Edouard Zarifian emphasizes the true therapeutic power of the physician himself and of the patient's circle, namely, family, friends, nurses, etc.:

> When using identical techniques, the relationship can or cannot be fully therapeutic. In order to have a relationship, there must be an interaction of two subjectivities. We could say in other words there must be a meeting of two desires: curing and healing. (1999, p.125)

But, for the patient or his or her doctor, to notice a therapeutic effect is not the same as desiring it.

In *The Status Syndrome,* Michael Marmot (2004) describes how it is important for the health of the individual to have enough 'decision latitude' for his social and professional issues. This is also true for the medical decisions of the patient and of the doctor, and it may well influence the efficacy of the treatment.

We should not confuse individualized and personalized medicine. Scientific and individualized care has to be developed on evidence-based observations, and to be fully efficient they must be offered to the patient in a personalized therapeutic relationship. This view of personalized health care brings us straight to what Paul Tournier has called 'medicine of the person'.

Can medical informatics save the relationship?

Indeed, it may well be the informatics which will allow physicians to save, if not to rediscover, the doctor–patient encounter, which has often been sacrificed, and to practise even better, if they so wish, a medicine of the person. But doctors themselves, and most of all those who teach medicine and train tomorrow's physicians today, should rapidly become conscious of it.

Today, medical training has been mainly replaced by teaching medical knowledge. Physicians today can no longer memorize and update the whole amount of medical knowledge they need every day for their patients' treatment. We should therefore stop burdening the student's memory with information he or she can only rapidly forget, when the computer is much more able to fulfil this job. On the other hand, he or she has to learn to use his or her brain because of its innumerable capacities of associations, which exceed the most powerful computer. He or she should also learn to use his or her intuition and his or her ability to meet the person of the patient in order to share a real personal dialogue and not a computerizable communication.

The teaching of medicine should distinguish in each subject the basic knowledge to which the physician should always be able to have immediate access through his memory, and all the rest he should know about and be able to access through informatics, when needed. The teacher should above all give the example of a physician who knows how to gather information and have access to it and to medical techniques, and how to integrate them all in a personalized therapeutic process.

If misused, informatics can lead to a depersonalized medicine, in which scores are used, and guidelines and algorithms are applied without discrimination, for the benefit of the greater number but with no consideration of the person. Informatics can allow the physician, or even make it compulsory, to see more patients in a shorter time with the highest economic efficiency.

Such a tendency already happens in some hospitals with the development of video connections between the office of the doctor and the bed of the patient. The main benefit for the patient is to have the opportunity to get in touch with his or her physician when he or she feels it is imperative. However, there is a great danger in using the device to reduce the time spent with bedside visits, allowing to the doctor to 'take care?' of more patients.

However, well used, informatics can allow the physician to have more time for the encounter, as well as to allow him or her to have access to the most recent knowledge and its efficient management. Information provided at the very moment when needed is better assimilated than if it is looked for later, and it results in an efficient way of teaching.

Some details may also have to be taken in consideration. Turning the head to look at the screen breaks the visual contact with the patient much more than writing a few words on a record placed on the desk. This comment by a patient led me to make a hole in my office desk for a touch-screen and this has been greatly appreciated by the patients.

The challenge of the third millennium may be to manage with intelligence the abundance of information, and if the Internet represents a triumph of communication, it may well jeopardize real encounters. The mastery of technologies can allow spectacular cures as well as encouraging the patient to give up the sense of responsibility in his or her fight against illness.

Our medical schools are full of experts learned in scientific knowledge, often very specialized, which is important for each of them and for what they are meant to teach to the students. Nowadays we need teachers involved in clinical medicine, providing models of healing people, able to develop and to use in an intelligent way medical informatics and who demonstrate with their whole person what should and could be a therapeutic relationship in which dialogue does not give way to science.

But we should not wait any longer. It takes more than ten years to train a physician. Starting at the very beginning of his or her medical studies, the student should be made aware of and trained to that new approach if we wish them to remain the master and not become the slave of the fascinating development of medical sciences.

Conclusion

Retaining the person in medical science means achieving the capacity to include evidence-based individualized health care, apprehending the multiple facets of a sick individual and providing this in a personal relationship.

Evidence-based knowledge is gathered through objective procedures, focused towards a 'sick object', which appears as the sum of the characteristics of a suffering person. But the core of the person, covered with altered biological functions, can only be reached and helped through a true personal encounter, involving the whole person of the caregiver. This encounter is therapeutic and can also have true biological effects.

Such a medical attitude cannot be taught in the same way as medical knowledge. It is not sufficient to repeat that encounter is important and worth the time it needs if the teacher does not show that he is behaving this way with his patients and with his students. He must not only exhibit a sparkling erudition but also be true in his behaviour. This will be a difficult challenge, since medical activity involves more and more teamwork, bringing the student face to face with several intervening physicians, making it difficult to find among them a convincing identification model.

The finality of the medicine of the person is not only to get rid of the diseases restraining life, but to promote health, with the assurance to be in life, which means to be in the movement of the life.

In our Judaeo-Christian culture, the discovery and the meeting of the person of God may open a way for the doctor who feels the need to encounter the suffering person. It is what Paul Tournier has experienced, and the meaning of his testimony.

References

Buber, M. (1960) *Urdistanz und Beziehung.* Heidelberg: Verlag Lambert Schneider.

Fierz, W. (2004) 'Challenge of personal health care: to what extent is medicine already individualized and what are the future trends?' *Med Sci Monit 10,* 5, RA111–123.

Levine, J., Gordon, N.C. and Fields, H.L. (1978) 'The mechanism of placebo analgesia.' *Lancet 1,* 654–657.

Marmot, M. (2004) *The Status Syndrome. How Social Standing Affects Our Health and Longevity.* New York: Times Books, Henry Holt and Company.

Orelli, A. von (1974) 'Person and Medicine'. Lecture presented at the 24th International Meeting of Medicine of the Person, Bristol, 1974.

Tournier, P. (1940) *Médecine de la Personne.* Neuchâtel and Paris: Delachaux et Niestlé.

Zarifian, E. (1999) *La Force de Guérir.* Paris: Odile Jacob.

CHAPTER 4

THE BIBLE AND MEDICAL PRACTICE

John Clark

Introduction

Paul Tournier's skill in helping doctors and patients to understand the meaning of life and of experience was inspired by his reading of the Bible as a doctor. Most of his books originated out of the biblical studies that he led at the annual gatherings of the Medicine of the Person group that have been held since 1947. People, he believed, need to know the significance of their illnesses and of their lives and to receive help from medicine in this discovery.

The Bible shows inspired people seeking to understand God's plan but finding it slowly and making mistakes. It is vital not to depend only on one's own interpretation of the Bible but to study, meditate and pray with other people (Matthew 18:20; Tournier 1954, p.134). Tournier noted how study of the Bible together by the members of a medical team led by Dr Lechler in his clinic at Karlsruhe created an atmosphere of acceptance and love. Together with his eight psychiatrists, Dr Lechler spent a whole winter in Bible study, training his team. He then held a Bible study session weekly. The influence of the Bible study was clear in the daily morning meeting that the psychiatrists shared with patients. The patients were given a chance to express their feelings and to enter into dialogue. When anyone spoke in the assembly, it was impossible to tell whether it was a doctor or a patient who was speaking (Tournier 1986, p.38–39).

Paul Tournier's reading of the Bible was well informed and thoughtful. It is marked by the discernment of a scholar. His appreciation of the need for a believing and thinking attitude to Scripture acknowledged difficulties in interpretation but recognized a coherent pattern of revelation.

He would have agreed with Archbishop Rowan Williams' view of Scripture as the 'unique touch stone of truth about God' (Higton 2004, p.62). Tournier provided reasons for his interpretation of biblical passages and so offered a way of working with the biblical text that others might use according to their own insights.

The approach to the Bible, recommended by Tournier, is a thematic one. It begins by taking the questions raised by daily life and going to the Bible for an answer. Alone, man does not even know who he is or where his faculty of asking questions comes from. The Bible provides a reliable guide. 'When we view the whole wonderful, unique and harmonious panorama formed by the person of Christ, the Bible, and the history of the Church, the evidence that God has revealed himself is overwhelming' (Tournier 1967, p.195). The message of the Bible, taken as a whole, leads to the conviction that all this could not have been either imagined or experienced without the intervention of God.

Tournier took as a guide a remark made to him by Emil Brunner. 'Let us read the Bible thinking constantly of our daily lives, and let us live our lives thinking constantly of the Bible' (Tournier 1954, p.18). The Bible is unparalleled in its richness and also totally human. 'The Bible is the book of the drama of life, and for us doctors, acting as we are all day long in that drama, it is of absorbing interest' (Tournier 1954, p.18). The language of the Bible is that of image and myth that touches the person more directly than the language of intellectual discussion. Its idiom is anecdotal; it is an experience, a personal truth.

The Bible is also strikingly realistic. It shows people as they actually are, with all their greatness, doubts, aspirations and vileness. 'Doctors will be interested to find that even feigned illness is described in the Bible (II Sam. 13:1–22)' (Tournier 1954, p.19). The realism of the Bible explains its contradictions. The Bible reveals the contradictory character of the human heart. It manages to grasp only a part of the truth. Among several examples, Tournier notices that James says that temptation does not come from God (James 1:13), while, in the Lord's Prayer, Jesus bids us to pray not to be led into temptation (Matthew 6:13) (Tournier 1954, p.19).

Biblical themes
THE NATURE OF GOD AND OF THE HUMAN PERSON
The Bible reveals what God is and what the person is. 'What is a person? It is man in so far as he becomes adult, freed from himself because

dependent on God, assuming full responsibility for himself before God' (Tournier 1954, p.122). Everywhere in the Bible people, touched by the divine dialogue, find their true dimension (Tournier 1957, p.172). It is a book of choice that sets people face to face with the supreme choice that determines all other decisions in life.

Tournier's books contain a precise picture of the character of God. He is the God who created and who governs the world in all its details. He is both omnipotent and perfectly good despite the apparent denial in the existence of evil and suffering. God rules over the destinies of people and, at the same time, leaves them free to disobey. God is absolutely sovereign (Tournier 1954, p.157), and great beyond the measure of our comprehension (Tournier 1967, p.61). The creation is an expression of God's love (Tournier 1966b, p.72; 1954, p.42). God governs the physical world (Tournier 1966b, p.183) and his purpose is worked out, not only through obedience, but also through disobedience (Tournier 1966b, p.93). God is everywhere, and at the same time, present in a particular place (Tournier 1968, p.43). He loves us individually and knows us by name (Tournier, 1957, p.169). He upholds us and speaks to us. His patience is without limit (Tournier 1968, p.200). He is interested in all that we do (Tournier 1964, p.10). No secret is hidden from him (Tournier 1965a, p.57). God is the author of all grace and the one true answer to human distress (Tournier 1962b, p.200). His love is unconditional (Tournier 1962b, p.192). He is a personal God who makes himself known (Tournier 1967, p.196).

According to the Bible, people are placed in a harmonious environment and provided through self-consciousness with a quality of life related to the life of God. In spite of the divine plan, people often think in a way that displays half-formulated ideas of an opposition between God and life so that God is seen as a brake limiting life. People claim to live their lives without the restrictive authority of God when, in fact, the truth is the other way round; God alone enables us to live to the full (Tournier 1954, p.140).

GRACE AND GROWTH

God's covenant with his people in the Old Testament sets the stage for the perspective of the Bible. The covenant marks the involvement of God in history. God's intervention gives to history its significance (Tournier 1954, p.76).

In the New Covenant, or New Testament, the perspective widens to include all humanity. The original covenant in the Old Testament and the historical life, death and resurrection of Jesus Christ provide the key to the meaning of the Bible (Tournier 1954, p.79).

Tournier saw Christ as unique in history and outside the limits of psychology (Tournier 1967, p.195). His life is inconceivable within the limits of classical psychological determinism.

The gospel of Jesus Christ is a gospel of growth. It aims at a development more complete than can be conceived by psychology confined within the limits of nature. All Christ's calls to detachment are accompanied by promises that point to their true meaning.

The surrender, demanded by the Christian life, Tournier saw as evidence of the compatibility of Christianity and psychology. God wills our development but also calls for the self-sacrifice necessary to obtain it.

Psychology helps people to follow the difficult road of renunciation. Faith recognizes this renunciation as a divine law and allows itself to be led by God and to rely on his support. 'The aim of psychology is the moral autonomy which men try hard to achieve, and the revelation of faith is that it is when one abandons oneself to Jesus Christ that one attains inner freedom' (Tournier 1968, p.209).

The Bible is a reflection of God's care for every person (Tournier 1954, p.123). God knows and calls us by name. It is not possible to achieve integration of the person unaided. One 'needs an integrating force, the Holy Spirit, and a supernatural guide, the Biblical revelation' (Tournier 1954, p.131). It is very important to read a biblical statement in its context, to know who is talking and to whom the words are directed before attempting to understand the meaning of a conversation or of an incident (Tournier 1962b, p.24; cf. Tournier 1967, p.129).

GUILT AND RECONCILIATION

Either we expect to win life on our own account or by faith in the grace of God. Apart from grace, one is left faced with a choice that is at once necessary and impossible (Tournier 1954, p.232–333).

The conscience of every sensitive person tells him or her that there is an absolute moral law. At the same time we must accept the reality of our own infidelity to it. This is the dilemma from which a way out must be found (Tournier 1954, p.234).

Tournier saw the solution in a personal encounter with Jesus Christ. The teaching of Jesus Christ is not an ethical system that can be carefully observed in order to free us from guilt (Tournier 1962b, p.120). It reveals something as always lacking, namely, our righteousness.

Christ not only forgives. He restores the insufficiency that is missing; and so life can become positive and free from anxiety (Tournier 1954, p.234).

The cross of Christ, and not individual effort, is the way by which fallen man is reconciled to God. Guilt deprives people of freedom. It is God who takes the initiative in obliterating guilt. The obliteration of guilt is free because of the sacrifice of Christ on the cross. The sacrifice of Christ accords with the deeply ingrained feeling, recognized by psychology, that a price has to be paid for sin. Christ does not become guilty. He accepts the consequences of our guilt. God provides the expiation that releases people from the vicious circle of guilt, sin and further guilt. If God has taken full responsibility for sin, it follows that there are no conditions attached to his love. Salvation is no longer a search for a perfection that cannot be found but a personal encounter with Jesus Christ. 'Remorse is silenced by His absolution. He substitutes for it one single question, the one He put to the Apostle Peter: "Do you love me?" ' (Tournier 1962b, p.187). Christ's solution to the problem of sin springs to life at the moment when one recognizes one's total incapacity to get right with God through the observation of a limited morality. Moralism often slips back into Christianity so that people seek salvation by their own effort and so pretend to be more virtuous than they are. According to the Bible, moral conduct is the spontaneous result of inner transformation by the Holy Spirit (Tournier 1967, p.151).

Dialogue with God always springs from an individual encounter. God's method is one of personal call. When anyone commits himself unreservedly to the way of loyalty, purity, self-surrender and the love of Christ, he transforms the atmosphere around him (Tournier 1962a, p.160).

Relevance to medical practice
TRANSFORMATION OF ATTITUDES
The value of the biblical perspective, Tournier believed, is that it radically changes our attitude towards the events of life. What matters is not whether they constitute success or failure but rather what they signify in God's purpose. This attitude engenders strength and independence in the face of people and events, even at times of the greatest failure. It is based on the conviction that God is working in everything for good of those who love him (Romans 8:28) (Tournier 1954, p.82).

An illness raises questions of two distinct kinds: (i) there are scientific questions about the nature and the mechanism of the illness, its diagnosis, aetiology and pathogenesis; (ii) there are also spiritual questions about the meaning of the illness (Tournier 1954, p.16). Tournier asked how doctors might practise a humane medicine without a religious faith. Unless doctors are convinced that their life has a meaning, how can they approach the questions of patients about human destiny? In cases of incurable illness, the patient expects the doctor to share in his suffering, accompanying him right to the end: 'He wants us to help him to live notwithstanding, and to help him to die. That seems to me to sum up the whole of medicine – helping men to live and to die' (Tournier 1954, p.179).

People suffering from the most difficult experiences can often find a solution only in faith:

> Of the meaning of things, the meaning of sickness and cure, of life and death, of the world, man and history, science tells us nothing; here it is the Bible that speaks to us. For this reason the study of the Bible is as valuable to the doctor as the study of science. (Tournier 1954, p.16)

Sometimes a doctor may help his patient deeply by a sincere declaration of his own faith. The patient may find a verse from the Bible the only relief. Tournier recalled a remark of Dr Alphonse Maeder 'that the doctor must learn to handle his Bible as he handles his pharmacopoeia' (Tournier 1954, p.184).

Tournier led the Bible studies at the annual conferences of the Medicine of the Person until, in later years, other doctors shared the task with him. The Bible studies were given at the beginning of the morning sessions. They were concerned with topics, investigated at the conferences, such as guilt, loneliness, strong or weak reactions, finding one's place in life or coming to terms with old age.

Tournier felt that the Bible studies gave a particular orientation to his daily medical practice, as they did to the work of the doctors who heard and remembered them. Tournier recalled, after many years' experience, in 1972: 'I have found deep joy in explaining the Bible to doctors of our time, in stressing the correspondence between our faith and the call of our vocation' (Tournier 1972b).

Tournier's voice resonated with enthusiasm and a lively intonation as he delighted over some new insight into the meaning of a biblical passage and its relevance to the life of a doctor. Points were often emphasized by gesticulations of his arms, as seen in the photograph overleaf.

His exuberance, enthusiasm and profound knowledge of the Bible were always clearly in evidence.

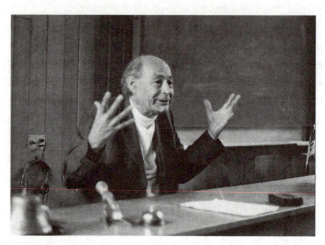

A typically expressive gesture during a bible study at the Medicine of the Person Conference in Bossey, 1973

Tournier observed that from the biblical perspective, faith, vitality and life are interrelated. Life means communion with God and death separation from him. The father says to the elder brother, in the parable of the Prodigal Son: 'This brother of yours was dead and has come to life' (Luke 15:32) (Tournier 1954, p.148).

Tournier noticed that it often happens that the re-establishment of faith manifests itself in a recovery of physical vitality. Where there is mutual love and understanding, vitality and psychological health are advanced. Tournier was sensitive to the mystery of suffering.

In spite of all the light thrown upon them by the Bible, the problems of pain, sickness and death remain for us an impenetrable and overwhelming mystery; here and there we can find in the Bible contradictory witness, answering to the varying experiences of believers before a problem that they do not understand. But the Bible itself does not claim to solve the problem. It lives it with us (Tournier 1954, p.222).

The identity of the patient has sometimes to pass through difficult crises and the experience of failure. Tournier believed that there is an inner development of the person that only affliction seems capable of producing. This inner growth of the patient, Tournier felt, also influenced him. He recalls the memory of patients facing sickness, bereavement, conflicts and failures and how the doctor and patient have always found a common bond as they carried the burden together.

> I remember too how I have seen them change through suffering, and how that has impressed me and changed me as well. It is true that the changes were not necessarily the ones that either they or I expected but I think that I can say that most of them gained by their experience as well as suffering from it. (Tournier 1982, p.15)

Experience shows that when suffering comes it brings us closer to Christ in his suffering (Tournier 1954, p.242). God does not send or will suffering, but the biblical view is that suffering is a school of faith (Tournier 1954, p.202).

FACING DEATH

Tournier was second to none in his commitment to relieve suffering and to heal the sick. But he realized that this is a temporary expedient. Life can be understood only in the light of eternity. 'This is why we feel ourselves to be "sojourners and pilgrims" on the earth (I Pet. 2:11); as Christians we know that "our citizenship is in heaven" (Phil. 3:29)' (Tournier 1954, p.203).

Death is a blessing from God. 'Through it we inherit eternal life in a world where "neither shall there be mourning, nor crying, nor pain any more" (Rev. 21:4)' (Tournier 1954, p.204).

Tournier was convinced that to accept death it is necessary to have faith in the resurrection. The Bible promises the resurrection of the whole person (Romans 8:11). In *Learning to Grow Old*, Paul Tournier wrote of the resurrection:

> I know that I shall retain my personal identity; and it is a fact here below, in personal fellowship, in the person-to-person relationship when it is true, that I find a foretaste of heaven. (Tournier 1972a, p.237)

The bodily resurrection of Christ is proof of this affirmation (John 20:27–28). In the resurrection, Jesus retained his identity. Our identity and communion with Jesus and with one another will be fully realized in the resurrection. Mary Magdalene recognized the risen Lord when he pronounced her name. Initially she had supposed that he was the gardener (John 20:15) (Tournier 1972a, p.237).

MEDITATION AND PERSONAL INTEGRATION

Tournier found in meditation a bridge between Christian faith and personal living. As a general rule, he did not see patients before nine o'clock in the morning (Tournier 1967, p.178). He allowed at least an hour a day for the practice of meditation. This, he acknowledged, meant giving up activities that he used to think of as essential (Tournier 1966a, p.215). Occasionally he would spend a whole day in meditation in the silence of a wood, a meadow or in a monastery (Tournier 1966b, p.217).

In an interview in 1984, Tournier was asked about his first experience of meditation. He replied, 'Trying to listen to God for a whole hour and hearing nothing at all' (Tournier 1986, p.14). At the end of the hour, however, one thought came into Tournier's mind; that he should continue the practice of meditation for a few days.

> Did this thought come from God? I don't know. Today I am persuaded that it did, in seeing what happened in my life. Not that for nearly forty years I have been faithful in meditation, far from it – but that, what has been most fruitful for me has come from it. (Tournier 1972b)

Tournier believed that the integration of the person is accomplished in meditation. To meditate is to be guided by God into self-discovery (Tournier 1954, p.133). Meditation is open in two ways, towards God and towards practical life. 'A single word received in meditation can transform a person's whole life, turning it into a great adventure' (Tournier 1966b, p.215). Meditation brings order into life, provides a point of reference and a goal towards which to direct attention. It involves a change in the person that conforms to God's plan. 'It leads him into the integration of contradictory tendencies which were hitherto tearing him apart. It is the entry into the deeper level which is called in the Bible metanoia (repentance)' (Tournier 1965b, p.63). Meditation has two aspects. It enables one to perceive clearly both one's own faults and one's vocation (Tournier 1966a, p.265). It is by listening to God that one is enabled to recognize the problems that are blocking contact with other people (Tournier 1986, p.40). Tournier often began his meditation by reading a passage from the Bible. He wrote down any thought that came to him in meditation, or any action to be taken. He believed that in meditation he could often find the solution to a problem that seemed insoluble. 'Meditation makes us independent of events by making us dependent on God' (Tournier 1967, p.185).

Problems often have their origin and stimulus outside the field of consciousness. Through meditation, one is enabled to appreciate more accurately the working and influence of the unconscious. A contraction of the field of consciousness takes place when a powerful tendency opposed to the moral values of the person makes itself felt within him or reveals itself through actions disapproved of by his conscience. The memory of these guilty feelings, or actions, is repressed from the field of consciousness. The repressed memories and tendencies reappear as dreams, unsuccessful actions, phobias, neurotic symptoms, paralyses or functional disorders. The more successfully that one is able to be honest with oneself, the more clearly one sees oneself; the contraction in the field of conscience begins to give way. One may then realize how often a conscious virtue arises from an unconscious fault.

> I strike my dog because he has been disobedient. But when I consider this during my meditation, I realize that in reality I was annoyed with my wife because of a remark she had made to me, and which at the time I had pretended to accept, when in fact I had not accepted it. (Tournier 1966a, p.250)

It is possible to experience not only a pathological contraction but also a pathological expansion of the field of consciousness. People readily take up attitudes to others, the hidden motives for which arise from the unconscious. These concealed motives spring from feelings like jealousy, self-centredness or the wish to cover up faults. The expansion of the field of consciousness leads to a spirit of criticism. People who are the most indulgent with themselves are the most critical of others.

In his recent book, *Living Love*, Dr Jack Dominian also speaks of the need to appreciate unconscious influences as they affect interpersonal relationships. 'By intuitive moments of insight, we render the unconscious conscious and accept what belongs to us and what is our responsibility' (Dominian 2004, p.94).

The complete opening up of the personality in a spirit of repentance, Tournier believed, leads to an enhanced mutual sympathy. A person who conceals distressing memories, remorse and private convictions also reveals in all his relationships a reserve that is intuitively felt. This reserve becomes an obstacle to personal relationships. On the other hand, all who meet the person who has confessed his sins feel at ease with him and so contact at the level of the person is the more easily achieved.

OTHER FAITHS

Tournier felt that faith involves a commitment to find a solution, not only to the problems of individuals, but for those of society as well:

Christian experience first of all restores the human person and then spreads out from person to person until it transforms society. Christ, after preaching to thousands, concentrated his attention upon a few disciples. It was to this handful of men that he confided the enormous task of taking his message to the ends of the earth. God's message throughout all of history has been one of personal calls. He calls a Moses or a Francis of Assisi, a Paul or a Karl Barth, to a life of rugged obedience, from which self-discipline all their spiritual, social and political ministry flows forth. (Tournier 1962a, p.163)

Tournier believed that there are two things that go into the making of a doctor: great scientific competence combined with a great heart (Tournier 1986, p.81). He preferred not to speak of a specifically Christian medicine. Science provides knowledge of the mechanism of things. The Bible speaks of their meaning. 'I do not believe that there is a Christian medicine distinct from ordinary medicine. What the Bible teaches about nature and about man is true for the whole of medicine' (Tournier 1954, p.35).

Doctors are able to create a bond that transcends the barrier between different denominations or even different religions: 'I have had contacts with Islam, and I have been able to gauge the possibility of uniting not only Christians, but also Jews and Moslems, in a spiritual view of man' (Tournier 1986, p.81).

Tournier appreciated the sincerity of people of different faiths or of no faith. He was clear about his own position that the intimate God, the friend ready to enter into dialogue, is Jesus Christ. He believed, as the Bible indicates, that God guides not only Christians but also people of other faiths or those of no faith. Divine support is not reserved exclusively for believers. Jesus spoke of the care of God for all people without discrimination. God prefers to grant his support to people who are conscious of their weakness rather than to the self-satisfied and the proud. For Christians, Jesus Christ is God incarnate:

But other people who profess a different religion, or those who claim to have none, stand to benefit equally from his mediation. God accomplished the reconciliation of humanity to himself. Our only privilege as Christians is of knowing it and proclaiming it. (Tournier 1966b, p.222 cf. Tournier 1978, p.56)

Discussing the search for divine inspiration, Tournier noticed how often fervent believers have been mistaken, like the people who crucified Christ or those who persecuted heretics at the time of the Inquisition. He spoke of Gandhi, who listened attentively to the 'still, small voice' (Tournier 1972a, p.155). Tournier recounted a conversation that he had with an Islamic leader in Tehran:

> We spoke there, Muslims and Christians together, of this spiritual part of life which is common to all men. It is a spiritual need that underlies all of our explanations, all dogmas and of the particular rites of each religion. (Tournier 1973, p.5)

Later, in *The Violence Inside*, Tournier wrote:

> It seems to me that it is Islam especially which has retained the sense of the sovereignty of God over the whole of human life, over social and economic life as well as the life of the individual. This is what gave their special flavour to the discussions that I had with Islam in Tehran. (Tournier 1978, pp.172–173)

Tournier tells how in Japan he was taken on a visit to some Buddhist temples. One Japanese doctor in the group commented that he had read all of Paul Tournier's books translated into Japanese and discovered there the third dimension of medicine. Tournier records the words of the doctor:

> I realized that in every sick person there is not only a psychological perspective, but also a spiritual one; and that there is a reciprocal relationship, as there is between body and soul, between the physical – the domain of classical medicine – and the propositions of religion. (Tournier 1986, p.50)

Conclusion: the two hands of medicine

Clinical practice had convinced Tournier that neither reason, nor science, nor the instincts, are themselves adequate guides to life. He worked to reconcile psychology and faith in a manner that prevented psychology from leaving a patient aware of his problems but without an understanding of how they might be resolved. He believed that faith, when spontaneous, could strengthen the will. He noticed that modern psychology has demonstrated the impotence of the will when it is not supported by imagination, in other words by faith in the psychological meaning of faith (Tournier 1967, p.95).

Tournier spoke of the medicine of the person as having two hands, the hand of scientific competence and the hand of personal communication. These two hands must be joined in prayer, a sign that one is listening to God, acknowledging his sovereignty and seeking his aid (Tournier 1978, p.192). In line with Tournier's appreciation of meditation is Rowan William's conviction that theology originates in worship, not in the seminar room (Short 2003, p.33).

Tournier was ahead of his time in his recognition of the coherence of knowledge. He drew attention to a view, now widely accepted, that science gives answers to factual questions, for example that the earth revolves round the sun because the sun exercises an attraction upon it. It does not explain why there is a universal law of gravitation. 'Faith alone replies because Someone has given the universe all its laws in order to fulfil His purpose thereby' (Tournier 1967, p.27). Religious belief is concerned with questions about the meaning of life in all its joys and sorrows and in its finite character.

The writings of Paul Tournier show how he discovered, in a biblical faith, an appreciation of experience that satisfied his understanding as a person and as a doctor and that enabled him to help his patients, and the vast numbers of people who read his books or heard him speak, to gain an awareness of the meaning of their existence and of their significance, one for another, in a manner that totally respected their freedom of thought and decision.

An aspect of whole person medicine involves the recognition that one's relationship with another person goes beyond what is said. What is felt may be more significant than any word. People know instinctively whom they can trust. To meet Tournier was to recognize immediately that one was in the presence of a person of transparent sincerity; a man who, through his Christian faith and the support of his wife and of many colleagues in the Medicine of the Person group, had a firm anchor that he always found reliable. From this stable base, renewed daily in meditation, he exercised a ministry of Christian love that often helped him to understand the needs of another person in a unique way. Tournier had the highest regard for medical science and for psychiatric skills. He had a fine intellect, supported by extensive reading and a critical judgement that enabled him to develop coherent, intuitive and original approaches to a wide range of human problems. Underlying the whole of his work was a firm conviction, regularly tested at the frontier of medical practice, that it is through Christian faith that one's gifts reach their fruition.

References

Dominian, J. (2004) *Living Love.* London: Darton, Longman and Todd Ltd.

Higton, M. (2004) *Difficult Gospel. The Theology of Rowan Williams.* London: SCM.

Short, R. (2003) *Rowan Williams.* An Introduction. London: Darton, Longman and Todd Ltd.

Tournier, P. (1954) *A Doctor's Casebook in the Light of the Bible.* London: SCM.

Tournier, P. (1957) *The Meaning of Persons.* London: SCM.

Tournier, P. (1962a) *Escape from Loneliness.* London: SCM.

Tournier, P. (1962b) *Guilt and Grace.* London: Hodder and Stoughton.

Tournier, P. (1964) *The Meaning of Gifts.* London: SCM.

Tournier, P. (1965a) *Secrets.* London: SCM.

Tournier, P. (1965b) *To Resist or To Surrender?* London: SCM.

Tournier, P. (1966a) *The Healing of Persons.* London: Collins.

Tournier, P. (1966b) *The Adventure of Living.* London: SCM.

Tournier, P. (1967) *The Person Reborn.* Student Christian Movement. London: Heinemann.

Tournier, P. (1968) *A Place for You.* London: SCM.

Tournier, P. (1972a) *Learning to Grow Old.* London: SCM.

Tournier, P. (1972b) 'My religious vocation as a physician.' In P.E. Johnson (ed) *Healer of the Mind.* Nashville and New York: Abingdon Press.

Tournier, P. (1973) 'The doctor, the senior citizen and the meaning of life.' *Journal of Psychology and Theology 1,* 2, 4–9.

Tournier, P. (1978) *The Violence Inside.* London: SCM.

Tournier, P. (1982) *Creative Suffering.* London: SCM.

Tournier, P. (1986) *A Listening Ear. Fifty Years as a Doctor of the Whole Person.* Texts selected by Charles Piquet. London: Hodder and Stoughton.

CHAPTER 5

THE VALUE OF VALUES – DO THEY GO DEEP ENOUGH?

Martin Conway

The what and why of values

The little word 'values' has clearly become quite a buzzword in today's society. My *Guardian* newspaper one day had a large headline: 'Living our values', over an advertisement inviting its readers to look up its social, ethical and environmental report of the year. When I did, I discovered a longish list of paragraphs itemizing points and activities in a number of different fields, from giving priority attention to areas staff are concerned about, to activities in and for local communities and the transparency of the paper's own governance, but hardly a clear list of 'values' as such.

I look eagerly at the various manifestos of the political parties for the various elections to see if – and if so, in what way – the word plays a role there. Meanwhile, one organization with which I happen to be closely involved, the Oxfordshire Community and Voluntary Action (the equivalent of a county-wide Council for Voluntary Services), recently took the occasion of the appointment of a new Director to give time to considering OCVA's 'mission and values'. We came up with 'Our mission: Enabling a diverse voluntary and community sector to flourish in Oxfordshire', accompanied by a list of five 'values': *equality, professionalism, empowerment, flexibility* and *collaboration*, each with a short paragraph setting out what we intend and plan to be and to do in order to give life to these somewhat abstract words. I imagine many of you reading this will have comparable statements and lists supporting and guiding your own professional communities and obligations. Clearly the term 'values' is expected to indicate a number of important commitments, priorities and political and ethical judgements about the work we do and the ways in which we do it.

The term is therefore something of a 'catch-all'. The matters it points to are clearly of importance, yet highly variable in nature, as in the way they function. My *Concise Oxford Dictionary* (1964) and *Oxford Reference Dictionary* (1986) give definitions only of the singular word, which suggests that the widespread use of the plural is even more recent than I would have imagined. Yet I suppose it to be reasonably clear in educated circles that the word is aiming to hold together in ways that will be widely accepted, for instance:

1. Matters of both 'truth' (how things actually are) and 'purpose' (how we intend to help them become).

2. Things that matter to any one of us (e.g. courtesy, or speed of response) and things that matter to the total team or profession (e.g. honesty and trustworthiness).

3. Matters that crop up at different stages of our life (youth, middle-age, retirement) and in different professional and family life contexts, so that we can know them and rely on them to embody in some important way a sense of continuity in our lives, of worthwhile tradition, and of as near permanence as a changing society can allow.

Of course we can and often will argue about the precise meaning of one or more of these 'values' in and for many different contexts in our lives. Those identified by the different political parties will no doubt at points look very similar even as they indicate directions for action that we know the different politicians, eagerly asserting their faithfulness to these values, will in fact interpret very differently, even in sharply contradictory ways! The values set out in their manifestos are intended to serve as uniting themes in our discussions, also as uniting priorities in our corporate action, but will by no means always be so perceived by the very different people involved. So while they can on occasion be truly inspiring and hope-giving, they can also be pretty vague, not to say 'slimy' when they allow certain people to 'get away with' what in other circumstances might have been called evasions, or even lies. In almost any imaginable context, 'values' are set out as positives yet can also prove to have dangerously negative effects. At best they are a curiously abstract and general way of identifying things of high – some would perhaps say 'the highest' – importance to the professions and institutions that identify themselves by them.

Pressures from the surrounding society

Any such discussion of 'values' must of course take account of what is happening in the society and culture with which we are concerned. Writing in Britain, and aware of the extent to which the various societies of at least Western Europe – and increasingly no doubt the entire European Union – are sharing the conditions of both society and culture to which I here refer, I suggest that there are at least four fields of which any such discussion needs to be immediately aware. The following points are not intended to evaluate what is going on among us so much as to point out, as matters of fact, developments and pressures that none of us in Western Europe can entirely escape. No doubt other nations and continents would provide comparable, if hardly similar lists:

1.   Social and cultural changes sweeping us all along in their wake.

2.   The astonishing degree of individualism we take for granted.

3.   The inevitable awareness of the different histories, cultures and faiths of humankind.

4.   The future of the human race, as of the planet, depends on us all, not just on some.

These are dealt with in more detail below.

SOCIAL AND CULTURAL CHANGES

I have only to look at the toys and playthings that my grandchildren take for granted to know that the first decade of the twenty-first century is already shaping them, let alone me, in ways they will neither think of going back on, nor ever want to. Electronic toys, for instance, zooming around a floor controlled by a small hand-set, give our children a familiarity with things moving around them at high speed that will help them grasp what aeroplanes are doing up in the sky or spacecraft in the distant fringes of our galaxy, and condition them to expect such things as normal in a way that I am sure I never could have at their age! More seriously, current patterns of, say, alcohol or drug use among teenagers, with all the consequences of official disapproval, of lessons devoted to stern warnings about their dangers, of police activity in curbing or forbidding their effects, cannot but wake an entire generation up to the possibilities and risks of human activities of which, again, I for one was wholly and happily ignorant until well into my twenties or thirties.

Archbishop Rowan Williams' strong warnings about depriving our children of their proper, indeed necessary childhood freedoms – alike in his recent letter to the heads of the major political parties in the UK and in his profound essay on 'Childhood and Choice' in his *Lost Icons – Reflections on Cultural Bereavement* (Williams 2000) graphically illustrate the risks we are making our children and future generations run. Yet it is hard indeed to know just when key dividing lines are being overstepped or when what begins as play with an absorbing new toy grows into a propensity to evaluate relationships and priorities in ways that will deform countless personal and ethical judgements in later years. 'A world of timeless consuming egos, adopting and discarding styles of self-presentation and self-assertion, is a social as well as a philosophical shambles' (Williams 2000, p.49).

INDIVIDUALISM

Where people of other cultures, say in Pakistan or China, will almost always identify themselves as part of their extended families or clans, we take it for granted in Western Europe that an individual – at least over the age of compulsory schooling – will expect to be identified and treated as a unique individual in the first instance, with no attention being paid to her/his family or community background. We have of course our ways of noticing indications of level of education, of class, of level of income, etc., yet our society in its legislation and in its good manners is insistent on both allowing and expecting each person to behave and be taken for a unique individual whose choices and decisions are up to her or him in her or his own freedom. From what you wear or what food you buy, through to what sort of job you aim at or who you choose as a long-term partner or husband/wife, all such life-shaping decisions are seen as deserving, indeed needing, to be left to the person involved, and in no way taken for them. This affects virtually every area of life. So that even if one's family and communal background, one's education and later experience do all of course condition, shape and indeed limit what one grows into being, it is considered the height of ill-treatment to force someone in any way into taking a key decision in this way rather than that, even in the case of relatively trivial ones – except of course where legislation gives the police or other officers of state the power to constrain what an individual may be trying to do!

This stress, often taken for granted without any precise thought about it, is the more heightened by the relative affluence of our societies, or at least of the more successful within our societies. People in reasonably good jobs can afford to buy many, indeed often most, of the things they would like to enjoy and possess – from food to holidays, from housing to favourite pastimes outside and after work. So an individualist society turns readily into a consumerist society, in which people will insist on being totally free to make their own choices of what to buy, and will value their possessions almost more than their relationships – or are easily tempted to do so. Any such conditioning then in turn affects what we 'value', let alone the 'values' we hold as priorities or as being determinative of what we wish to aim at and become.

DIFFERENT HISTORIES, CULTURES AND FAITHS

I have been pointing to the peculiar characteristics of Western European societies, some of them shared with North America as a comparably affluent area, though it is in fact culturally very different in many ways. At the same time, one of the major effects of the 'globalization' that has developed so startlingly since the end of European colonialism in the 1950s and 1960s, is – and this alike in the more affluent nations and the poorer ones – that human beings are almost all at least aware that there are many other nations in our world, each with its specific history, people and culture – let alone language(s) – that others do not share. Thus we almost all know that we are 'one world', that we all belong in some inevitable way to a single planet. Moreover we are increasingly aware, in any part of this world, that we are in contact with at least some people originally from one or more different parts of it.

This affects people differently. On the one hand, say, farmers in Africa have become aware how strongly the agricultural markets of their own country, and therefore their own livelihoods, are affected by the prices of goods imported from other countries. At the same time, urban dwellers in the West are now experiencing in their own cities substantial populations of incomers from other parts of the world, including second and third generations who display quite new combinations of the culture and expectations of both their present homeland and of that of their parents or grandparents.

Very few of us can now live without some strong awareness of other peoples, other cultures, other expectations about the future of our one world. This affects, for instance, our view and experience of sports – virtually none of which is now limited to one nation – as it does of holidays, or of music, with a constant shifting of fashions and possibilities, increasingly diverse as different areas of the world come into play.

So also with regard to 'values': we may be aware of the kinds of things that matter for our own part of the world, indeed for our own communities, customers or constituents, but any such communities and groups will be becoming wider and more diverse, leaving more room for people of very different backgrounds. So we age-old British find it tricky to know how to share at depth with a range of other people from different backgrounds, and wait in hope for the time when they have become more fully 'integrated' into what we go on calling 'our society and its culture'.

In particular this is greatly affecting the major 'religions' (better to speak, with Wilfred Cantwell Smith (1978), of 'communities of religious traditions') from around the world. I live in Oxford, with its many historic Christian memories, yet now with a splendid new Arabian-style mosque along the road from my house, and lively groups of Buddhists and Hindus, as well as the long-established Jewish community, reminding all Christians and every citizen of Oxford that the world offers different choices also in the sphere of 'religion'. Just as we rather enjoy the mixture of different styles of music, even if some of us are better than others at appreciating these in their variety, or of different languages or forms of art, where few outside each major tradition feel at all readily at home, so also in matters of religious faith the consumerist knowledge that there are many different realities around the world and in our city make many of us the more hesitant to commit ourselves wholeheartedly to any one in a way that might exclude or lessen possible appreciation of the others.

THE FUTURE OF THE HUMAN RACE AND THE PLANET
The more threatening part of this same awareness comes from the environmental side, namely that the future of our planet, as a place on which it will be possible for living beings, including the human race, to go on living, is under serious risk if we insist on continuing to burn fossil fuels and to send greenhouse gases into the atmosphere. If and as we do, the age-old patterns of our climate will become ever more seriously disturbed. To put it over-simply, the human race will either sink together in a whirlpool of destruction that we have brought on ourselves, or we may be able to find ways of pulling through together – which can only come about if we do indeed all pull together in a total effort. This last option neither will nor can happen if we continue to behave either as if some people in high places will look after the problem while the rest of us

continue to do what we like; or if we continue to suppose that the lives of some matter considerably more than the lives of others. Any attempt to safeguard the interest of a few will only contribute more actively to the destruction of the whole. We are hardly yet at the point of voicing this often, but it is surely becoming steadily more apparent, even unmistakable.

These four developments discussed above all seem to me to condition in important ways our awareness and trust in the 'values' that we are so keen to list and discuss in professional and other circles. I suspect that in different ways these four areas of awareness make it increasingly difficult for our 'values' lists and convictions to grip as firmly as we would wish on the realities we have to handle.

Do they go deep enough?

Here I need to start writing like the Christian theologian I try to be. For as well as the factors I have listed above, with the implied critique that it is no longer good enough – if it ever was – for us Europeans to suppose that 'we know best', we need to look further into the roots and lasting reliability of what we commend as 'values'. Any such 'values' are unlikely to remain true and effective in a world constantly being thrust deeper and deeper into these complexities. It is going to become harder and harder to reach adequate points of common understanding and commitment to any values, unless we can establish just where they are rooted and grounded, and in what way this can remain trustworthy for each new generation.

This is where it is all-important for me, as for most 'religious' people (not that that term, undiscussed, can signify much that is readily identifiable these days), to realize and remember that humanity's basic affirmations and ground-rules over many, many centuries have come not just from among ourselves, but from those we recognize as lasting, in most cases permanent, 'authorities'. In India's many cultures and subcultures, these have been found in the Vedas, as in the Lord Buddha (and other, more recent, gurus); in pre-communist China Confucius used to be venerated as the reliable ancestor, though he clearly took many of his teachings from yet more ancient sources. In the Jewish–Christian–Muslim 'worlds' it is in the creator God, and prophets and teachers who refer all questions of their authority to that supreme and revealing, if never wholly known or measurable God, to whom reference for ultimate authority in all questions of human or indeed the planet's life is made.

So it will be no surprise if I point way back to the Ten Commandments of Moses, to the example and teaching of Jesus of Nazareth, to the messages entrusted to Mohammad and recorded in the Qur'an, as the origins and roots of almost all our trusted 'values' for today. This is not of course to identify everything that 'religious' people have said and done down the centuries as invariably right and reliable – far from it! Precisely because 'religion' is seen as all-encompassing, a matter of the highest truth and importance, people are the more tempted to misuse it – and when they do to cause the more horrible and confusing of misunderstandings, because they are betraying what are – and rightly so – expected to be truth-filled and reliable precepts.

Differences between the major religions

I have allowed myself to use the term 'religion' for this large and diverse field spanning many different cultures, yet of course the major religious traditions are by no means the same. Each has its own history, its own teachings, its own distinctive way of understanding the world and of advocating certain ways of behaving rather than others. We help no one if we try to claim that all 'religions' are the same. At the same time, and here again especially in the Jewish–Christian–Muslim 'worlds', whose traditions feed into and draw from one another's at more points than most of us are accustomed to recognize, the basic affirmations of God the Creator and of his purposes in creating the world as it is, with humankind 'in his likeness' and as his 'stewards', are essentially the same, even if our three traditions have disowned and misappreciated one another all too often, and all too cruelly, down the ages.

As a matter of historical fact, there can be no doubt that it has been the propensity of the different 'religions' to reject and fight one another that has been the strongest single factor in leading the peoples of Europe – and now of other areas too – to turn away from them, to reject their claims, and now to be looking for rather different 'values' by which to organize and raise the quality of the life and developments we share in. Any believing Jew, Christian or Muslim needs to be fully aware of this, and approach this whole subject with a proper humility, even repentance. For the ways in which people such as ourselves – in history and still today – can so easily identify our selfish hopes and wishes with God's purposes prevents these last, in the inevitably mysterious ways they can become known to humanity, from governing our fallible choices, decisions and teaching.

I learned long ago in the Student Christian Movement that any claim of a religious tradition to truth and profound meaning can never be taken as more than a hypothesis to be tested out. As soon as 'religion' becomes something imposed on some people by others it can all too easily become a witness to a false God. By the same token, religious 'obedience' is always essentially a 'pilgrimage': a shared journey of exploration and ever-deeper discoveries, leading into shared convictions about truth and goodness, yes, but which must never be taken to be wholly identifiable with God's wishes simply because 'I say so'! In a rapidly changing and developing world, the 'gap' between the basic awareness of God's love and purpose for us all as essentially God's gift, and the specific possibilities and decisions that each of us has to face in complex and changing situations, is always big enough for us to be able to make serious mistakes. Yet to say that is not to invalidate the appeal, at the basic level, that it is worth taking the trouble to search out, discuss widely, and feel one's ways towards the truly 'God-given' response and decision, rather than rush into the usual or widely expected or politically convenient decision. The sorts of question that our statements of 'values' are meant to address are still of the highest importance for the common life, so that it matters even more than we can readily know, actively to search out, rather than expect to be able readily to decide on for ourselves, the genuinely future-opening responses and actions that the situation may require.

As for the sensitive differences between the religious traditions, while this cannot become the place for a full discussion, the best single framework for regarding and handling them that I know, was drawn up in 1981 for the British Council of Churches in four apparently simple and linked 'principles for inter-faith dialogue' (British Council of Churches 1991):

- *Dialogue begins when people meet each other.* It is *persons*, not religions, not teachings, who can meet and interact. Even when people stand in very different cultures and traditions, friendship is always in principle possible. There is always something to be shared, some contact worth making.

- *Dialogue depends upon mutual understanding and mutual trust.* This may take time – it never comes very easily. And it may take the overcoming of many misunderstandings. But, like friendship, it can never be said to be totally impossible in principle. It is there to be worked for.

- *Dialogue makes it possible to share in service to the community.* People of faith know that they are called not just to live their own lives, but to devote time and care to their neighbours, not least those who are in any way disadvantaged or in difficulties. So a dialogue that is discovering mutual understanding and trust can be of great service to the people of a divided and fearful community.

- *Dialogue becomes the medium of authentic witness.* Yes, there are deep differences between our faiths and traditions, and we need – in God's good time – to open up to one another about these, and explore how they can be best appreciated and possibly resolved between us. It is only in established friendship that these can best be tackled in the hope of discovering that, far from dividing us, they can lead us into deeper and shared convictions to enlarge the service we can together give to the community.

The deepest and most reliable convictions

As a Christian, what matters most to me is to be able to see whatever I am handling as in some way related to the purposes of the creator God who has made himself known to humankind in the man Jesus of Nazareth. In that one life, as in the Jewish tradition and culture that helped to shape him, I believe that humanity has been offered the crucial experience of truth and of purpose in life, with both of these stemming in and from the God who created humanity and everything else in the first place. More-over, in the way Jesus lived, all of us in the human race can experience a life lived for the purposes of God, in service of what God wills for all people everywhere. Not a series of commands and recipes for 'getting things right', but a series of stories about human relationships, about finding new health where people could only see demonic powers or death, about living in the belief that God has a purpose for every single person and situation that can add up for each person too, in God's good time, to a life worth living and sharing for eternity.

This is why, for Christians, the Bible is the essential aid to living in love and truth and hope. Not because it tells us exactly what to do in our various heres and nows – it doesn't! But because it tells in many overlapping and always enlarging stories how God's gracious love and power has been sensed and followed out by different people in different situations, climaxing in Jesus' short but intense ministry in the time of Pontius Pilate, and in the beginnings of a tradition of Jesus-following lives and thinking in the records of people such as Paul, Peter, James and the John to whom the book Revelation was given. These all add up, including their manifold human varieties and complexities, to a single story of God and his purposes in leading the human race he created to serve as his stewards of the rest of the creation towards its true fulfillment. That single story in turn invites each of us to lead his/her own life story within its horizons, within its all-encompassing purposes and the moral qualities that best anticipate the fulfillment of those.

This side of death, each and every human being is bound to have endless questions to raise, as much about our present situations as about the complex yet recognizably 'single story' of God and his creation. These questions are seldom easy to 'answer', let alone easily 'answered' in our various behaviours, but are nevertheless an important gift to us worth exploring. Indeed, with regard to these questions the 'single story' of the Bible as read by Christians encourages its readers to believe it is always possible to work towards answers that will be right not just for ourselves but for all humanity. One key to that work, that exploration, is to look steadily and attentively not first for what I or we can do, but rather for what I or we are being given – no doubt by others around us yet in the final instance by God – as pointers, methods and tools for our next steps in the exploration and the pilgrimage.

Do our 'values' go deep enough ? If they are supposed to be self-sufficient, no – most unlikely. However, if they can be servants, not just of our own immediate hopes and intentions but rather of the purposes of God, as Christians have seen in Jesus, and not just for myself but for all my human neighbours in every walk of life and for the entire creation entrusted to our care, then maybe yes. I hope and pray that they can.

References

British Council of Churches (1991) *In Good Faith – The Four Principles of Interfaith Dialogue: A Brief Guide for the Churches.* London: CTBI.

Hawkins, J.M. (ed.) (1986) *Oxford Reference Dictionary.* Oxford: Clarendon Press.

Smith, W.C. (1978) *The Meaning and End of Religion – A New Approach to the Religious Traditions of Mankind.* London: SPCK.

Sykes, J.B. (ed.) (1976) *Concise Oxford Dictionary.* Oxford: Clarendon Press.

Williams, R. (2000) *Lost Icons – Reflections on Cultural Bereavement.* Edinburgh: T & T Clark.

PART 2

FAITH TRADITIONS AND MEDICINE OF THE PERSON

CHAPTER 6

THE CHRISTIAN TRADITION OF SPIRITUAL DIRECTION AS A SKETCH FOR A STRONG THEOLOGY OF DIVERSITY

Robert Atwell and Bill (K.W.M.) Fulford

Paul Tournier was a man of deep Christian conviction whose faith became the inspiration and springboard of his life and work. His theological roots were in the Calvinism of Geneva, but his mind and outlook were truly ecumenical. His medicine of the person, as the editors of this book (Chapter 1) and other contributors (e.g. Rüedi, Chapter 3) make clear, had a strong spiritual basis, but one that was never partisan or religiously exclusive. Indeed the distinctive feature of his approach was a meeting of the *person* of the doctor with the *person* of the patient in an open and inclusive encounter that was profoundly respectful both of the wide diversity of individual values and beliefs that he encountered, and of the different cultural and faith traditions that were the context of his clinical work.

Respect for diversity of values and beliefs as the basis of a 'liberal theology' has traditionally been contrasted with the 'strong theologies' of more dogmatic and fundamentalist creeds. There is indeed strength in such creeds. It is the strength of the ideologue, whether religious, ethical or indeed scientific. In this chapter, by contrast, we illustrate the resources for what we will call a 'strong theology of diversity' from the Christian tradition of spiritual direction. This ancient tradition combines, as Paul Tournier's medicine of the person combined, deep personal conviction with an intuitive openness to a spectrum of values and beliefs in those who declare their need for guidance and help in periods of transition, confusion, distress or mental disorder.

We start with a contemporary (though biographically disguised) story from pastoral care, the story of Sarah. We then describe some of the key ideas from the tradition of spiritual direction that stand behind the encounter between Sarah, her husband and their vicar. Much of the chapter is taken up with drawing out the richness of these ideas for the strong theology of diversity that, we believe, they embody. In a brief concluding section we return to the central and irreducible role of personal engagement and relationship, equally in pastoral and in clinical care, which is perhaps the enduring legacy of Tournier's medicine of the person.

The story of Sarah

Sarah was a woman in her mid-40s, happily married with three children, all in their teens. Having successfully undertaken a degree with the Open University, she had returned to paid employment. Apart from what at the time seemed a minor medical problem of moderately raised blood pressure, discovered during a routine medical check up organized by her new employer, she was thriving in every way. But then the unexpected happened: she became pregnant. The gift of a fourth child, even though unplanned, would normally have been greeted with joy, but given Sarah's recent medical history the news was cause for considerable anxiety. As the pregnancy progressed, it began to provoke major fluctuations in her blood pressure, which required two periods of hospitalization. After the second spell in hospital the consultant gynaecologist recommended the termination of the pregnancy, stating that Sarah's health, and perhaps life, were at stake. She and her husband were given 48 hours to think about it.

Both parents were committed Anglicans and, although not absolutist, in their view abortion was ethically wrong: the rights of an unborn child should be protected and upheld. Abortion represented the wanton destruction of human life. In some distress, not least at the pressure the medical profession were putting on them, Sarah went to see her vicar. Although she enjoyed a good relationship with him, she was also anxious about how he would respond to their dilemma. She desperately needed to unburden herself, and wanted someone to tell her what to do, but was fearful at what that person might say. In her vulnerability, she was open yet defensive.

The vicar listened with real empathy but, to Sarah's surprise, held back from telling her what to do. The questions he asked were open-ended and non-judgmental, enabling her to speak candidly about her situation. Together they looked at the various options, including talking about guilt feelings in relation to having an abortion. He suggested that they meet again the following evening, this time with her husband as an equal participant in the conversation. When they asked the vicar for his opinion he declared his antipathy to abortion but said that he saw his role not to tell them what to do, but rather 'to travel with them', and crucially, he said that he would support them *in whatever decision they made.*

In the event, Sarah did have the abortion. She believed it was the 'right' decision, and although it was something that filled her with sadness at the time, she never regretted it. Subsequently, as her vicar anticipated, she experienced an episode of self-recrimination and guilt feelings about the abortion. She asked for and he readily gave her absolution, and she received the 'laying on of hands', with prayer for the healing of her memories.

Spiritual direction

Reflecting on this story, the key point to note is that the language Sarah's vicar used (consciously or unconsciously) was one of *journey*, of *accompanying*. His talks with Sarah were directed not at producing a predetermined outcome but at building the quality and equality of their engagement as *persons*. He and Sarah were engaged in what, adapting Tournier's term 'medicine of the person', we might call 'pastoral care of the person'. In the terms of spiritual direction, Sarah and her vicar, and subsequently Sarah's husband, were involved in a *process of discernment*. We will return to what this means in detail later. But some of the obvious parallels between the process of discernment as reflected in pastoral care, and the process rather than outcome-oriented approach of Tournier's 'medicine of the person' in clinical care, include:

1. Listening – seeking to understand the particular needs and circumstances of that individual and why they had come to see you.

2. 'Staying with' – rather than giving answers ('this is right' or 'this is wrong'), working with the person to help them find a solution for themselves.

3.   Avoiding absolutes – whatever your own values, starting from maxi-
     mum sensitivity to the individual and the situation in which they
     find themselves.

Clearly a conservative Roman Catholic priest or a fundamentalist Protestant pastor in a similar situation might have responded differently, perhaps upholding an absolutist position, and as a result been more directive
in their counsel. Sarah's doctors, from their quite different perspective of
concern for her health, were equally directive in their advice that she
should have an abortion. At its best, however, the Christian tradition of
spiritual discernment is about process, the process of engagement of person with person, rather than prescribing outcomes. The ongoing practice
of spiritual direction, as we shall see, building on ideas and concepts developed and refined over the centuries in the Christian church, combines
a strong commitment to the highest moral ideals in tandem with the
greatest sensitivity in dealing with each individual, a sensitivity that hon-
ours a person's particular values and beliefs, and which relates to the particular concrete circumstances in which they find themselves.

   That the openness and respect for differences of values and beliefs at
the heart of spiritual direction is a basis for a strong theology of diversity,
rather than being a reflection of a weak 'liberal' compromise, is evident
not only in the rich texture of the theoretical concepts that underpin the
tradition, but also in the practical effectiveness of their outworking and
the quality of resulting pastoral care. In the remainder of this chapter,
therefore, we describe some of these concepts and illustrate their contemporary relevance, including the way in which, explicitly or implicitly,
they stand behind the encounter of Sarah with her vicar. They are:

- friendship
- self-knowledge
- a word of life
- direction
- compunction
- desires
- discernment
- healing.

We start with what to many may seem an unlikely concept in this context,
that of friendship.

FRIENDSHIP

Historically, the practice of spiritual direction emerged within Christian monasticism. During the fourth and fifth centuries thousands of men and women went to live for months, sometimes for years, in the deserts of Egypt, Syria and Palestine. They went to pray and to seek God. Great emphasis was laid upon the importance of personal discipline, silence and solitude, but paradoxically what monasticism spawned was a culture of charity and friendship. Ordinary people journeyed into the desert to seek counsel from the monks. Thus was born a tradition of holy conversation (if it may be termed so) in which a person engages over a period of time in prayerful reflection about their life with a fellow Christian, their 'director' (who may or may not be a monastic or priest but who has the role of wise counsellor). Together, they seek through a process of discernment the guidance of God. In the ancient Celtic Church such a wise counsellor was called a 'soul friend', a title that reflects the quality of engagement and trust that these encounters elicited.

Writing in the twelfth century about such 'spiritual friendship', the great Cistercian abbot Aelred of Rievaulx said:

> Medicine is not more powerful or more efficacious for our wounds than the possession of a friend who meets every misfortune joyfully, so that as the Apostle Paul says, shoulder to shoulder, they 'bear one another's burdens'... The best medicine in life is a friend. (Aelred of Rievaulx, transl. by Laker 1977, p.72)

Friendship is the unlikely concept to find at the heart of pastoral, and indeed clinical, care in contemporary practice. The relationship between minister/priest and individual members of his or her congregation, like the relationship between a doctor and his or her individual patients, is nowadays understood as requiring a degree of professional distance. This is perhaps one of the points on which Paul Tournier's close friendly relationships with some of his patients may sit rather uneasily with contemporary understanding of professionalism. On one occasion, for example, as Thierry Collaud describes (Chapter 11), he took one of his patients who was suffering from his existential questioning on a three-day hike in the mountains to help him deal with these problems! At the very least, this would be an unconventional approach in modern clinical or pastoral care, although it was consistent with the practice of his day. But the general point remains that in professional relationships boundaries have to be carefully sustained according to the mores of the time, and inappropriate forms of intimacy avoided.

In the tradition of spiritual direction, however, friendship (understood in the specific sense of a meeting of souls) is a prerequisite. Moreover, there is an entirely appropriate sense in which, if a pastoral encounter is to be fruitful, it *has* to be intimate. Friendship and intimacy, as these ideas are understood within the tradition of spiritual direction, were essential in the meeting between Sarah and her vicar. There was indeed a meeting of souls: remember that Sarah and her vicar both started from a point of deep ethical concern about abortion. As a consequence, in the meetings between them the emphasis was on seeking the will of God, and that seeking was mutual. In the Christian tradition the 'director' and the 'directee' are both seekers: both are partners in a spiritual conversation, a current of spirituality. Indeed in the Christian understanding the true director in any encounter is understood to be the Holy Spirit. Any attempt on the part of the so-called 'director' to make the 'directee' dependant on his or her own insights, rather than reliant on the Spirit's guidance, is eschewed because a person must be encouraged to take responsibility for themselves and make their own decisions.

SELF-KNOWLEDGE

Spiritual direction then as now is essentially about the encounter of the self with God, and inevitably this process includes facing oneself. In this understanding, self-deceit is self-destructive. Gregory of Nyssa, a theologian and bishop writing in the early fourth century, sounds a remarkably contemporary note in this respect:

> Our greatest protection in this life is self-knowledge so that we do not become enslaved to delusion, and end up trying to defend a person who does not exist. This is what happens to those who do not scrutinize themselves. They look at themselves and what they see is strength, beauty, reputation, political power, an abundance of material possessions, status, self-importance, bodily stature, a graceful appearance and so forth; and they think that this is the sum of whom they are. Such persons make very poor guardians of themselves because in their absorption with externals they overlook their inner life and leave it unguarded. How can a person protect what he does not know? The most secure protection for our treasure is to know ourselves: each of us must know ourselves as we are, and learn to distinguish ourselves from what we are not. Otherwise we may end up unconsciously protecting somebody who we are not, and leave our true selves unguarded.' (Gregory of Nyssa, *On the Song of Songs*)

Sarah's unexpected pregnancy and the precarious nature of her health was an enormous shock to her and to her husband. The prospect of an abortion challenged many of their deeply-held values and beliefs, and forced them to think through (discern) where they stood in relation to the Anglican Church with which they identified so strongly. Ultimately they negotiated the crisis well and attained a deeper self-knowledge. Far from being diminished by the experience, their lives and marriage were deepened by what happened.

A WORD OF LIFE
In monastic circles, friendship and self-knowledge were closely allied to the desire for 'a word'. It is in the desert that we encounter for the first time the figure of the *abba* or *amma*, charismatic holy people who exhibited wisdom beyond their years, who knew God and themselves well. People would seek out these holy men and women, to share their silence, and to ask them for advice and guidance. The phrase, 'Speak a word to me, father/mother', recurs again and again in the literature of the Desert Fathers and Mothers. This was spoken not in expectation of 'an answer to a problem', or a theological explanation or rationale; nor was it 'counselling' in any kind of conventional way that we might recognize today, or a kind of dialogue in which various points were debated. Instead 'a word' was part of the relationship, something that would bring life and hope to the disciple if it were received.

Words and shared silence, and healing through words and silence, were similarly important in the story of Sarah and constituted good pastoral care. In mental health practice too, there are many 'talking therapies', as they are often called. But the early monastic concept of 'the word of life', like the concept of spiritual friendship understood as a meeting of souls, has a deeper resonance close to the central feature of Tournier's medicine of the person; namely, healing through relationship.

DIRECTION
The particular meaning attached to 'the word' as healing through relationship is connected with a further feature of spiritual direction; namely, that the notion of 'direction' in 'spiritual direction' has nothing to do with telling someone what he or she should do. It is rather about self-discovery through relationship.

Again, this was crucial in the story of Sarah. The decision to have an abortion that she and her husband came to was *their* decision. They came to it through a process of self-discovery that was enabled by their talks with their vicar, and informed by the medical knowledge of their doctors, but was nonetheless their own mature decision. This, we believe, was crucial to their ability subsequently to carry their decision through to a healing outcome. Other couples might have come to very different decisions. It is not the outcome but the process that is crucial. *Any* decision that had not been 'owned' by Sarah and her husband, whether to have an abortion or to risk taking her pregnancy to term, would have left a gap that could have proved impossible to heal.

Here, as in all spiritual direction, much devolves upon the integrity and maturity of the vicar/pastor. Few have made this point with greater contemporary relevance than one of the great ascetic women of the desert, the fourth-century Amma Theodora. She said:

> Such a teacher ought to be a stranger to the desire for domination, vain-glory, and pride. One should not be able to fool him by flattery, nor blind him by gifts, nor conquer him by the stomach, nor dominate him by anger; but he should be patient, gentle and humble as far as possible; he must be tested and without partisanship, full of concern, and a lover of souls. (Ward 1975, p.83)

COMPUNCTION

In monastic writing we encounter various references to the *gift of tears*, and something that is often associated with it, namely, *compunction of heart*. These puzzling references are key terms in the vocabulary of early Christian spirituality, and although no longer fashionable, are closely linked in substance to contemporary understanding of the potential for self-knowledge and spiritual growth through crisis.

The experience of sickness, marriage break-up, failure, bankruptcy, depression, addiction, redundancy or bereavement, can precipitate profound spiritual upheaval in a person's life. In such circumstances people of faith draw upon the rich resources of their spirituality and beliefs in their struggle to cope, and may become more religiously observant, rather than less so. Some may react negatively, finding themselves coping with the disappointment that their faith did not after all immunize them from the traumas of life, and end up questioning it. Equally traumatic can be the experience of having to make major decisions in life, particularly when (as with Sarah) they descend without warning. Such experiences can challenge a person's cherished values and interrogate their underlying motives and desires.

We habitually use the word 'crisis' for such events in our lives, and often the word carries with it a negative connotation. But the Greek (and Biblical) word from which our English word 'crisis' derives is wholly positive: *krisis* means simply judgement. As its etymology suggests, a crisis is a time of judgement and decision that yields self-knowledge, psychological healing and discernment.

The origin of the word 'compunction' is similarly interesting. It was a medical term of the ancient Roman doctors – *compunctum* – designating attacks of acute pain, but gradually it came to be applied by Christian monks to pain of the spirit. As our English word 'puncture' suggests, the Latin term came to designate a pricking or uneasiness of conscience, a remorse born of penitence. It described a radical openness to God, which made possible moments of profound disclosure when falsity and self-deceit are stripped away, and the human heart is pierced by a perception of the truth that will ultimately set the person free. The ancients conceived of men and women each having a reservoir of accumulated tears inside them resulting from the grief and sorrows they had never expressed. Compunction released those tears. The crisis experiences were painful but ultimately liberating. They signalled healing, much as the pain of a cyst that is lanced by a doctor brings relief and signals the beginning of healing. Thus tears were not seen as a problem (as so often in our own culture) but as a gift, evidence of the spirit of God moving in someone, releasing them and, as was the ultimate outcome with Sarah and her husband, healing their hearts.

DESIRES

Are our desires our enemies or our friends? Sarah's story, from the perspective of some fundamentalist positions, demonstrates the suspect nature of all human desire: she sacrificed her unborn child. Sadly, many religious people (of all faiths) have been taught that our desires as men and women are dangerous obstacles to the accomplishment of God's will, and should be suppressed. At its best, however, the tradition of spiritual direction, as exemplified for example by no less a figure than St Augustine (354–430), is characterized by an entirely positive attitude toward desire.

One of the texts on which St Augustine liked to meditate was, 'O Lord, all my desires are known to you' (Psalm 38:9). In company with other early Church Fathers, he was realistic enough to know that it is a fallacy to think that you can find total or final fulfilment of all your aspirations in this life. Boredom and restlessness, he taught, are universal phenomena. They are not something to be ignored, much less escaped from or anaesthetized, but rather entered into because the experience has the potential to project us into the embrace of God in whom alone is peace and stability. As Augustine wrote memorably in his *Confessions*, 'Our hearts are restless till they find their rest in you, O God.'

It is fashionable to caricature Augustine as a grumpy, negative, killjoy. But the dominant words in his spiritual vocabulary were in fact delight, desire and love. Augustine recognized in these strong, confusing (and sometimes frightening) energies, hallmarks of our common humanity. What is it we desire and long for? What do we delight in? What do we seek? What is it we want? What do we love? He recognized that these questions are central to all people's lives, and it is as we wrestle with them that a way forward in life emerges. Human beings are created with needs, longings and desires, and in the words of the Psalmist, the God who 'searches us out and knows us' is well acquainted with them. The problem, according to Augustine, lies with us: we know neither ourselves, nor what we want, nor the God who invites us into intimacy. 'If I knew myself,' he argued, 'I would know God' (*Noverim te, Domine, noverim me*) (St Augustine, *On the Trinity*).

Generations of people have been taught in the name of religion that feelings are to be mistrusted and ignored. They have been encouraged to devise various strategies to control, tame or suppress them. But in Augustine's view, to seek to be immune from our desires is to seek to be sub-human. Our desires are something positive, natural and God-given, not a problem to be solved or overcome. They emerge from deep places within us. As Pope Gregory the Great wrote a century after him, 'The language of souls is their desire' (Gregory the Great, *Moral Reflections on the Book of Job*). Desires go deeper than feelings, which are often transient, surface phenomena. They are not something we create or arouse in ourselves but rather, as Augustine realized, something that we discover. Our desires are an expression of the deepest truth about ourselves, and form, as they formed for Sarah and her husband, the very agenda of spiritual direction.

DISCERNMENT

Desires, then, in the tradition of spiritual direction, are recognized as key factors that shape our lives and our life choices for good or ill. But if 'for good or ill', how should we evaluate the difference 'in quality' between them, particularly given that they are not always as transparent as they may appear? The answer to this question brings us to the concept at the heart of spiritual direction, the concept of *diakrisis*: discernment. As the Greek reveals, the term is derived from the word for 'crisis' and means literally, 'right judgement' – or as an old Christian prayer has it, 'to have a right judgement in all things'.

On this subject, the greatest treatise without doubt is by St Ignatius of Loyola (1495–1556), founder of the Jesuits. His *Spiritual Exercises* represent a compendium of advice on spiritual direction and the 'discerning of spirits', to use his characteristic phrase. The text, first published in 1548, was not meant to be read, but was designed as a guide to assist the spiritual director who would lead the directee through an extended retreat, often as long as 30 days. Ignatius' teaching has spawned a whole tradition of prayer and discernment, particularly within the Catholic Church.

Philip Sheldrake, in his important study *Befriending our Desires*, has provided a contemporary study of Ignatian spirituality and its implications for our understanding of healing. He encourages us to seek a relationship with our desires, indeed to 'befriend' them. He promotes a holistic view of life, and a correspondingly holistic view of ourselves. Sheldrake urges that no one should ever say that a desire is irrelevant to the process of their spiritual growth. He writes:

> As a process, discernment enables us, in the first instance, to be aware of and to accept the full range of desires that we experience. From this starting point we are slowly led to understand the way in which our desires vary greatly in their quality. Certain desires, or ways of desiring, if we follow them through, will tend to push towards a dispersion of our spiritual and psychic energy or a fragmentation of our attention, experience and personalities. Other desires seem, rather, to promise a greater concentration of energy and a harmonious centredness. What is sometimes initially confusing is that the less helpful or healthy desires appear to be more strikingly attractive because they make us feel good. In other words the direction and potential of our desires is not always immediately self-evident. (Sheldrake 1994, p.79)

HEALING

As it evolved, early Christian thought was greatly influenced (both positively and negatively) by the all-pervasive climate of neo-Platonism in the ancient world. One negative example of its influence can be seen in a recurrent antipathy to the body. The recovery of a more balanced, holistic view of what it means to be a human being is one of the achievements of twentieth-century thinking, and it corresponds to the fundamental belief of Christianity that all of life is the gift of God. In this perspective there are no water-tight compartments: the physical, emotional, social and spiritual well-being of human beings are closely interconnected. It is the whole human person that is made in the image of God. In the words of St Irenaeus (c.130–c.200), another wonderful voice from the early Church: 'The glory of God is a human being fully alive' (Irenaeus, *Against the Heresies*).

The corollary of this teaching is that everything that undermines life, that diminishes, destroys or denigrates it, is inimical to God. In this perspective, caring for our bodies (as opposed to indulging or abusing them) and for those of our neighbours is as much a spiritual endeavour as the nurture of our souls. This is why the New Testament uses the term 'healing' both for physical healing and for the broader salvation that it proclaims that Jesus Christ brings. The Gospel of Jesus is a gospel of love (Raven 1949). The healing of bodies, minds and memories, the reconciliation and restoration of relationships, all of which went hand in hand in the story of Sarah, are integral to that gospel, and consequently continue to shape the Christian understanding of health and disease, and inform its own distinctive tradition of spiritual direction.

Conclusions

In this chapter we have described some of the formative ideas in the Christian tradition of spiritual direction and illustrated their application, by reference to the story of Sarah, in the context of contemporary pastoral care. Our aim has been to indicate the extent to which Paul Tournier's medicine of the person, although based on an open and respectful engagement with the diverse values and beliefs of individual people, is still set firmly within a great faith tradition. Spiritual direction, like medicine of the person, is not concerned to prescribe this or that 'solution' from a pre-set menu, be it spiritual, scientific or ethical. Like medicine of the person, it is based on relationships between people, mutually respectful of their differences of values and beliefs, and working together in a shared process of healing.

Paul Tournier's medicine of the person, like all models of the healing relationship, is to some extent a child of its time. In particular, its strongly dyadic nature requires, as other contributors to this book indicate, translation in the context of such contemporary health care developments as team working (Chapter 12) and preventive medicine and public health (Chapter 13). Yet on the one hand with the recent resurgence of religious and ethical fundamentalism, and on the other, a positive explosion of scientific advances in medicine (some of which like reproductive technologies and transplant surgery challenge our deepest received intuitions about our shared human nature), there has perhaps never been a time when the central lesson of Paul Tournier's life and work was more urgently needed. The dogmatists on both sides, those for whom inductive science is *the* answer equally with those for whom this or that received religion or ethical system is *the* answer, will dismiss medicine of the person with its essential openness to differences of values and beliefs as hopelessly liberal and outmoded. We believe, to the contrary, that set against the backcloth of two thousand years of spiritual direction, Paul Tournier's medicine of the person provides a much needed and wholly contemporary sketch for a strong theology of diversity.

References

Aelred of Rievaulx, *On Spiritual Friendship*, II, 12; translated by Mary Eugenia Laker SSND (1977), Kalamazoo, MI: Cistercian Publications.

St Augustine, *On the Trinity*, IX, 18; *Corpus Christianorum: Series Latina 50*, 293; translated by the author.

Gregory of Nyssa, 'Homily 2 "On the Song of Songs"'; J.P. Migne (ed.) (1857–1866) *Patrologiae cursus completus: Series Graeca 44*, 763; translated by the author.

Gregory the Great, 'Moral Reflections on the Book of Job'; J.P. Migne (ed.) (1844–1864) *Patrologiae cursus completus: Series Latina 75*, 1028; translated by the author.

St Irenaeus, *Against the Heresies*, IV, 20, 6; *Sources Chrétiennes 100*, 640; translated by the author.

Raven, C.E. (1949), *Jesus and the Gospel of Love*. London: Hodder and Stoughton.

Sheldrake, P. (1994) *Befriending our Desires*, London: DLT.

Ward, B. (transl) (1975) *The Sayings of the Desert Fathers*. Oxford: Mowbrays.

CHAPTER 7

PERSONHOOD IN HEALTH CARE: JEWISH APPROACHES

Claire Hilton and Michael Hilton

> There can be fewer vocations more interesting than that of seek-
> ing to understand the human person. (Tournier 1957, p.45)

Paul Tournier was an advocate of a 'medicine of the person' combining
medical knowledge, respect for the individual and religious insights.
Coming from a strongly Christian perspective, Tournier's views cannot
be translated directly into Jewish terms. But many elements of his writings can be interpreted through a Jewish perspective, including values
such as the importance of repentance. However, in the twenty-first century the identity of a Jew is based on far more than religious experience
alone. Personal identity within Jewish communities is complex, only
partly linked to the Jewish religion itself, and influenced by other cultural, historical, social, psychological and spiritual factors.

Thus in a health care environment it is not possible to understand the
needs of an individual Jew purely on the basis of knowledge of the religion. Huge diversity exists within the Jewish community in synagogue
affiliation, beliefs, knowledge and culture. All of these may influence a
Jewish patient's response to illness and the attitudes of a Jewish health
care professional.

Jewish spirituality

The following two quotations are worthy of consideration:

> After dinner my wife and I...to the Jewish Synagogue...But,
> Lord to see the disorder, laughing, sporting, and no attention, but
> confusion in all their service, more like brutes than people know-

ing the true God. (The Diary of Samuel Pepys, 14 October 1663, on the festival of the Rejoicing of the Law)

What most Western thought takes as spiritual rhetoric is largely foreign to traditional Jewish discourse. (Hoffman 2002, p.6)

These quotations serve as a warning to those approaching the topic of Jewish spirituality in a religion whose adherents often emphasize deeds more than faith. Lawrence Hoffman defines Jewish spirituality as 'our way of being in the world'; a religion which involves responsibilities that move beyond the house of prayer, into the home and out into the world. Some Jews find a spiritual meaning for their lives through devotion in prayer; others through the weekly Shabbat (Sabbath), a day of rest; some through the rhythms of Jewish home life; others through the cycle of the festivals; some through social action; others through Zionism; some through Jewish food; others through Jewish culture; or through the major events of the Jewish life cycle; or through any combination of these facets of Jewish life. This huge variety becomes understandable if we consider Daphne Wallace's definition of spirituality, when she writes about *Spiritual Aspects of Dementia* (Wallace 2004, p.215): 'Spirituality can be described as a search for that which gives meaning and identity to a person's life and the wider world'. This is a wide definition. Its manifestation will be different for each individual. Person-centred care must take account of whatever that individual's spiritual needs are. Wallace argues that attending to spiritual needs means to focus on 'being' rather than 'doing', but with Jewish spirituality both aspects must be regarded as equally important.

Setting the context: the British Jewish community

British Jewry remains a small and changing community. With total numbers estimated after the 2001 census at 267,000 (Office for National Statistics 2001), it is mainly located in the larger cities, in particular London (56%), Manchester and Leeds. Within London, the largest communities are in the north-west of the metropolitan area, especially the Borough of Barnet. Home to almost one in five British Jews, there is huge Jewish religious diversity within this small area. The most visible *Haredi* (ultra-orthodox) Jews, with men mainly dressed in traditional black clothes, is small, comprising only 8.5 per cent of the entire Jewish community, and living mainly in Barnet and Stamford Hill in London and in Salford in

Greater Manchester. With the small size of the British Jewish community and its patchy locations, many non-Jews in Britain may never actually meet a Jewish person, and misunderstandings about the community, and the use of stereotyped beliefs and images is not uncommon. For Jewish people living in smaller communities, where health care staff have little experience of working with Jewish people, the implications for staff gaining a good understanding of Jews as individuals are huge. With the high number of staff from abroad, especially front-line nurses who are frequently from countries in Africa and Asia with very small Jewish communities, this situation is further compounded. Small matters of communication, often overlooked but frequently overheard in the health care environment, such as the use of colloquial phrases 'touch wood' or 'cross your fingers', both alluding to obtaining good luck from the cross of the crucifixion of Jesus, may be disconcerting or even offensive to Jewish patients.

British Jewry has certainly changed from the early twentieth-century model of assimilation and acculturation. Perhaps with the growth of the multi-cultural society in Britain the Jewish community has become more confident in itself, with the flourishing of Jewish day schools since the 1980s and more frequent displays of Jewish identity such as the wearing of a scull cap (the *kippa* or *yarmulke*) in public areas, a practice not just restricted to orthodox Jews. Yet these positive changes may be tempered by the effects of the political climate in the Middle East. The relationship of the Jewish community in Britain to Israel has recently been summarized as 'attached to Israel, but ambivalent about its policies' (Cohen and Kahn-Harris 2004, p.44). However, the effect of the political tensions are such that synagogues in Britain have their security rotas, and religious services and Sunday school classes take place in buildings with trained security personnel on duty. Jewish day schools have their security guards, and on school outings boys from orthodox schools will be likely to wear a secular baseball cap rather than a *kippa*, identifying them as Jewish. The Community Security Trust is an important and extremely active charity within the Jewish community working closely with the police, government and other organizations on matters relating to antisemitism and security, and providing trained security volunteers for Jewish communal events and institutions. Thus confidence is undermined by fear.

Synagogue membership

Eighty per cent of Jewish people in Britain pay an annual subscription to a synagogue. A recent survey by the Board of Deputies of British Jews showed that 80% of British Jews are synagogue members, and of these, 57% are mainstream Orthodox, 20% Reform, 9% Liberal (Progressive), 8.5% Haredi (ultra-orthodox), 3.5% Sephardi (from southern Europe, North Africa and Asia) and 2% Masorti (Conservative) (Cohen and Kahn-Harris 2004, p.17).

For some, their synagogue membership may correlate closely with their beliefs and practices, such as belonging to an orthodox or reform synagogue. However, for many this is not the case. Some maintain membership of a particular synagogue because they have paid their burial insurance subscription to that institution for many years, and changing synagogue may affect their burial rights in a particular cemetery, possibly close to the grave of a loved one. For many older people this is a crucial issue; religious beliefs and practice may change with time, but synagogue membership may not. Even the unaffiliated may want a Jewish funeral.

Some people convert to Judaism, others marry outside the faith. They are more likely to be members of Reform or Liberal synagogues, raising an additional dimension for the healthcare professional who may be caring for a Jewish patient with non-Jewish close relatives. Others join a synagogue because they feel comfortable with that particular style of religious service – the music and chanting, the balance between the use of English and Hebrew – largely unrelated to their beliefs in God or their religious practices outside the synagogue. Whereas some will attend services daily or weekly, many others in British Jewry attend twice a year, on the High Holy days – on Rosh Hashanah, the New Year and Yom Kippur, the Day of Atonement – days for prayer, reflection, repentance and forgiveness, ideas also central to Tournier's philosophy. Whereas a synagogue may have a regular Shabbat morning congregation of 200 worshippers, almost the entire membership may request seats for the High Holy days, possibly ten times that number.

Despite this not being a straightforward issue, the diversity of synagogue membership may give health care staff some clues to a patient's religious requirements. However, synagogue affiliation is not currently recognized as important information by the National Health Service (NHS), either in the Department of Health's minimum data set collection, or in data that are usually recorded on the identification front page of a patient's hospital notes. Whereas Christian denominations are recorded,

e.g. Roman Catholic, Church of England etc., within minority religions
the same process of identifying subgroups is not followed, thus missing
out on a vital but basic opportunity to encourage staff to think about
religious diversity and identify patients' individual care needs.

The Jew as an individual within a community

The Jewish religion recognizes the importance of both the individual and
the community. The acknowledgement of the importance of the individual and the place of the Jew within the community is intimately linked
with the individual's thinking, identity and behaviour, as the following
quotations (from the early centuries of the Christian era) illustrate:

> One man only was at first created in the world, to teach that if
> anyone has caused a single person to perish Scripture imputes it to
> him as though he had caused a whole world to perish: and if any-
> one saves the life of a single person Scripture imputes it to him as
> though he had saved a whole world... Also to proclaim the great-
> ness of the Holy One, blessed be He: for when a man stamps many
> coins with the same seal they are all alike; but the holy One,
> blessed be He, has stamped every human being with the seal of
> the first man, yet no two are exactly alike. Therefore, everyone is
> required to say, 'For my sake was the world created.' (Mishnah
> Sanhedrin 4:5)

> Hillel says Do not separate yourself from the community... Do
> not judge your fellow until you have been in his position. (Mish-
> nah Avot 2:5)

More modern interpretations of this theme emphasize the importance of
self-searching and repentance, in a way of which Paul Tournier would
have approved:

> Rabbi Simcha Bunam of Pzhysha (died 1827) taught: Everyone
> must have two pockets, so that he can reach into the one or the
> other according to his needs. In his right pocket are to be the
> words 'For my sake was the world created' and in his left 'I am
> dust and ashes.' (The Reform Synagogues of Great Britain 1985,
> p.357)

A Jew who escapes an accident or recovers from an illness has the opportunity to recite a special blessing of thanks to God. This blessing (known

as *gomel*) is not said privately but in the synagogue when the community are present. The individual acknowledges that the benefit of recovery is to restore him or her to the community of which he or she is part.

However, in the twenty-first century, the relationship of a Jew with the community may not be straightforward. For many, being part of the community may be regarded as a spare time activity, analogous to a hobby. A Jew is likely to identify more closely with the community at some times than at others, or with some aspects of religious life more than others. In the modern world we frequently compartmentalize different aspects of our lives, and this can lead to a dissociation between religion and the secular world. In Paul Tournier's words 'the tension that always exists between the person and the personage is one of the conditions of our life, and we must accept it' (Tournier 1957, p.83): people respond and behave differently in different environments and social situations. In a health care setting, for example, a Jewish staff member may not want to reveal his or her Jewish identity to a Jewish patient, for fear of being asked to prioritize the patient's care needs or give them preferential attention because of their communal identity and responsibilities. The converse may also be true within a small community: the patient may not want a Jewish care worker to know of their problems because of who else they might know in the community and fears that their predicament may not remain confidential. In these ways both patients and practitioners respond to the conflict between traditional community and a secular world which usually demands that we do not bring our individual cultures into our professional relationships.

The modern tendency to professionalize everything is destructive of community in other ways. The duty of the physician to heal and of the patient to consult a doctor is deeply rooted in ancient texts, and the practice of medicine has always been a valued occupation within the Jewish community. Acknowledgement in the wider community of the role of Jewish physicians goes back more than a thousand years. The most famous of all was Maimonides (Moses ben Maimon). Born in Cordoba, Spain in 1135, Maimonides became the principal rabbi in Cairo and physician to the Court of Saladin. His medicine was his means of earning his living because he refused to make money from his religious scholarship. Today there are still plenty of Jewish doctors, but if you visit a Jewish care home you are likely to find that the staff is entirely non-Jewish. Caring has become professionalized. The community donates money and others do the work. The sense of a community really looking after each other in the traditional way is not there. In this respect, the personal has been lost from these aspects of care. Despite this professionalization of health care, most synagogues have volunteer care groups who informally help and support those who are unwell within their communities.

Belief in God

It has been argued that the British Jewish community may in reality today be an ethnic minority rather than a religious group (Cohen and Kahn-Harris 2004). Even among those Jews who consider themselves 'religious', their belief in God may be partitioned off from aspects of secular life. It is interesting that Tournier worked towards an understanding of the person from within his Christian religious framework, whereas Freud, a secular Jew, mainly approached the issue from outside a Jewish religious framework. Unlike for many Christians, God is not a normal topic of conversation within the Jewish community. Prayers tend to follow set texts and the tradition of personal and spontaneous prayer is ignored by many. Thus at times of crisis the Jew comes face to face with questions of doubt and questions of faith that are unfamiliar. Confronted by suffering, both Jewish patient and Jewish carer may not know where to look for guidance.

Belief in God may be separate from an individual's knowledge of Jewish laws and traditions, both of which may influence attitudes and behaviour. Contemporary medical ethics (see later section), an important and specialized area of Jewish law, offers carefully and well-developed answers for many of today's dilemmas. But precisely because it is a specialized area, it may be unknown to many Jews. A Jewish individual's knowledge of the rights and wrongs of decision-making and ethics in medical care may be more based on attitudes of the surrounding majority culture, in particular of Christianity. The individual's knowledge and practices may also cause confusion and surprise in a health care setting when patients prioritize their family traditions and their own interpretations rather than traditional Jewish teaching and 'text-book' descriptions of the Jewish religion (see Case Study 7.1). Despite this, some knowledge of the Jewish religion remains important if health care professionals are to understand the care needs of their Jewish patients. The website of the Jewish Hospital Chaplaincy Services (www.jvisit.org.uk), edited by a rabbi and written for hospital staff, appears readable, informative, concise and accurate.

Case Study 7.1: Using an individual's Jewish traditions rather than religious law in health care

Mrs A. lived in North West London and was 75 years old. She was admitted to hospital as a social care emergency with police involvement when the neighbours were concerned about the arguments and crying coming from her home. She had been physically, financially and emotionally abused by her daughter and mentally disabled granddaughter with whom she lived. Although a member of an orthodox synagogue since childhood, she had not attended any synagogue activities for years. Because of the financial abuse, her pension had been stopped and she had no money whatsoever. As she was beginning to become more confident in a geriatric ward, the occupational therapist wanted her to visit the hospital shop as part of rehabilitation. However, a proud woman, she would not accept money from ward funds for this purpose. It was December, and the time of the festival of Chanukkah. There is a tradition of giving money on Chanukkah. So, in discussion with a Jewish staff member the occupational therapist made a card that said 'Happy Chanukkah, please accept this Chanukkah gelt from the Ward' and enclosed £5. The patient was delighted.

Home and family life

The family is often the means through which the Jewish individual becomes part of the community. As much as the synagogue, the home is the spiritual centre of Jewish religious practice. Traditionally, synagogue attendance has not been compulsory for orthodox women. For many others, family practices at home such as eating the Friday evening Shabbat meal together or attending the family seder service and meal on the eve of Passover may be their Jewish focus. In the home as well, inherited family traditions may be a stronger component of Jewish life than religious ritual practice. So a Jew who always eats traditional food on various festivals – such as milk-based foods on Pentecost (Shavuot), apples dipped in honey to signify a sweet year on the New Year, fasting on the Day of Atonement, and so on – may not request kosher food during a hospital admission.

The emphasis on Jewish home and family life adds to the disorientation that can be experienced after a sudden or unplanned hospital admission. For example, an orthodox Jewish man who wears *tefillin* every morning at home, may feel embarrassed about wearing a leather box on his head and arm in a hospital setting. Orthodox Jewish visitors may have walked from home to the hospital to visit a sick family member on the Sabbath and may well have come without refreshments or money, because of definitions of work that include travelling, carrying and spending money. Such situations require awareness and sensitive handling by health care staff.

For an observant Jew, visiting the sick is not just paying a social call, but an important religious duty. The visitor is expected to attend to the patient's practical needs and to pray for his or her recovery. Even for the pious, practical help takes precedence over theological speculation, as the following story from the end of the third century of the Christian era demonstrates:

> Rabbi Hiyya bar Abba fell ill and Rabbi Yohanan went in to visit him. He said to him: 'Are your sufferings welcome to you?' He replied: 'Neither they nor their reward.' He said to him: 'Give me your hand.' He gave him his hand and he raised him. (Babylonian Talmud, Berakhot 5b)

Twentieth-century Jewish history

> All that we have lived through and felt in the past is inscribed in us, and helps to make us what we are today. (Tournier 1957, p.70)

Another aspect of the individual that may affect their acceptance and compliance with health care is their personal life experience, a concept also central to Paul Tournier's ideas. Still in Britain today are many Jews who were refugees or survivors of the Nazi era. Although they are not alone amongst ethnic minority groups who have witnessed, experienced or survived genocide, their experiences relate directly to their Jewish backgrounds. Typically, they have spent their working lives achieving as much as they can. Activity helped to suppress distressing thoughts of their past. However, in older people activity may be reduced, there is more time to think and reflect, and this may cause distress. For some survivors, authority figures such as health care staff or people in uniform may be a symbol of suspicion and persecution rather than help and support. For those who experienced concentration camps, loss of self-control under daily life circumstances would likely have been their demise. Sixty years on, issues around adjusting to illness in old age, when maintaining control and autonomy over ones actions and life may become daily challenges, may cause particular difficulties for survivors. Similarly, previous trauma may influence health care decision-making in the context of increasing physical illness and disability. Psychologically, the more painful the situation, the more the patient may be reluctant to speak of it, and the more important it is to know something about the history of the period in order to tactfully enquire (see Case Study 7.2).

Case Study 7.2: The importance of personal and community history in health care

An elderly Jewish woman had a chest infection and was admitted to a medical ward of a hospital. She was thought to be depressed and was referred to the old age psychiatry team. She had come to England from Vienna in 1938 at the age of 16 years as a refugee. Her daughter, she said, now lived in Vienna but never invited her over. 'How do you feel about going back to Vienna?', she was asked. She replied that she could not go as the memories would be too painful for her. Perhaps her daughter never asked because she recognized and understood this. For the patient, the schism in her family relationships in the context of her personal history was of paramount importance. Difficulty coping with this was undermining her wellbeing and enjoyment of life. For the old age psychiatrist, the challenge is to help this patient come to terms with her history and the reality of current family circumstances, and to help her cope better with her predicament.

Medical ethics

Social, cultural, historical and psychological factors also interact with Jewish medical ethics as well as the medical situations faced by patients and care providers. With the diversity of the Jewish community already acknowledged, it may well be under the heading of Jewish medical ethics that conflict is most likely to arise. Unless a Jewish practitioner is aware of the specifically Jewish origins of his ethical stance on some issues, inappropriate advice may be given. There are specific guidelines on certain medical issues, in particular relating to life and death issues, such as abortion, fertility, contraception, organ transplants, termination of nutrition or artificial life support and potentially life-threatening forms of medical treatment. Many rabbinic opinions on these and other issues can conveniently be consulted on the Internet, with the caveat that individual opinions are not necessarily authoritative and patients may well therefore wish to take advice from their own rabbi. Patients and relatives may appreciate consultation between the doctors and the rabbi, regardless of their degree of orthodoxy or beliefs (see Case Studies 7.3 and 7.4). If the patient does not have a rabbi, the Jewish Hospital Chaplaincy Services may be approached.

Case Study 7.3: Rabbis and doctors

It was Yom Kippur (Day of Atonement – 25-hour fast day – no food or drink permitted) and a large congregation were in the Reform synagogue, many of whom were fasting. An elderly, frail-looking woman collapsed, and was carried out to the first aid room by the large gentleman who had been sitting next to her. Several congregants who were doctors, including eminent physicians from the local university teaching hospital saw what had happened and followed them out. She had by then recovered to a certain degree and this group of doctors all tried to encourage her to have something to drink. She refused until someone whispered in her ear 'the rabbi says you must have something to drink!'

Ethical issues affect Jewish hospital staff as well. For example, an orthodox Jewish doctor may be reluctant to sign cremation forms for a Jewish person, as cremation is forbidden in orthodox practice, although permitted by the Reform and Liberal synagogues in Britain.

At least one aspect of British medico-legal guidance impinges directly on the care of Jewish patients. There are current debates on the confidentiality ethics of informing hospital chaplains about the religions of in-patients in hospital. Whereas, for majority-population religions, the chaplains can pay regular visits to wards and talk to nurses to see if any patients wish to see them, this is not a practical option for a minority religion like Judaism (see Case Study 7.5). Other recent controversies like having single-sex wards, may also affect orthodox Jews where specific dress codes relating to modest appearance may be important. The provi-

sion of a 'chapel' rather than 'interfaith prayer room' may also tend to discourage Jewish people from using a prayer facility within a hospital
setting, because of the specific Christian connotations of the word
'chapel'.

Case Study 7.4: The family of a dying Jewish patient

The family of a severely ill Jewish patient in an intensive care unit consulted their rabbi in a distressed state. They reported that the patient, although unable to speak, had indicated to them by gestures that he did
not wish to be fed or treated. He subsequently lapsed into a coma. They
went on to explain that medical staff were asking their permission to
discontinue treatment. They felt they were being asked to make a
life-or-death decision which was beyond them, and which might be
contrary to Jewish traditions on reverence for life. The rabbi held discussions with them and with the medical staff, explaining that while
Judaism teaches the sanctity of life, it does not require the undue prolongation of a life of distress or pain. The ethical issue of consent to
treatment was also explored: the patient, unable by that time to give
consent, appeared previously to have indicated to the family his decision to refuse further treatment. The medical staff accepted that having
taken everyone's views into account, the decisions about treatment
rested with them. The patient was allowed to die peacefully.

Case Study 7.5: On a paediatric ward

My eldest son was three weeks old when he was admitted to hospital.
He had pyloric stenosis, a blockage at the lower end of the stomach.
This condition has a tendency to occur more frequently amongst
Sephardi Jews, and requires urgent abdominal surgery. The diagnosis
was made early on Friday morning, but because of long theatre lists, the
surgery had to be postponed to take place on the Sabbath. Of course
the operation had to be done, but the timing made the situation even
more anxiety provoking. Then he got a wound infection and a chest infection and required a course of intravenous antibiotics, and we were

both in hospital for two weeks. Medically it was all very traumatic. I was desperately trying to establish breast feeding, but I was not the patient and was not entitled to food on the ward. If I had wanted kosher food, then all my food would have had to have been brought into the hospital, as kosher meals are only for patients. As it was, when I did go to the canteen I was told that I was a visitor, and any vegetarian or non-meat food was for staff, and I had to wait to the end of the meal session to be served if there was any left. None of the ward staff told me that if you wanted to see the hospital Jewish chaplain you had to request that as he did not automatically visit the wards. I still remember, and much appreciate, a nice member of our synagogue bringing me 'ethnic' Jewish food – bagels, smoked salmon and cream cheese – on a Sunday morning.

The health care situation

Most of what has been written here is based on experiences within British Jewry and the NHS. Because the issues include the interactions between staff and patients, and many of the staff may also have different sociocultural backgrounds, the contents may not be directly transferable to other countries. For example, belief in God is generally considered to be more widespread in the population in the United States of America than in Britain, and this may affect the dynamics of staff–patient interactions on religious matters. On the other hand, a recent report on British Jewry (Cohen and Kahn-Harris 2004) emphasized parallels between Britain and other diaspora communities. In Israel, however, there are certainly other sociocultural aspects interacting with the religious identities of Jewish people. The importance of the subtle interplay of social factors interacting with the individual person was recognized by Tournier (1957). Medicine has to be set in the context of people's social, psychological and cultural needs, understanding and beliefs. This chapter has explored the great diversity of issues that may arise between Jewish patients and health care staff within this framework.

Learning points
CASE STUDY 7.1
Jewish traditions rather than *halacha* (religious laws) may be more significant in the lives of some Jewish people, and can be useful therapeutic building blocks.

CASE STUDY 7.2

For this patient it was her previous history, as a Jew, which was a cause of her distress, not dilemmas created by the religion itself.

CASE STUDY 7.3

Reform as well as orthodox Jews may have concerns about the health/religion interface, possibly on the basis of incorrect knowledge about religious principles. In this case, it was perfectly appropriate for the doctors to encourage her to take fluids and for her to take their advice without the rabbi's intervention. She however wanted rabbinic advice.

CASE STUDY 7.4

In some circumstances, a rabbi can be a valuable part of a health care team, helping relatives and medical staff understand ethical issues, and developing an acceptable response to a situation.

CASE STUDY 7.5

A degree of understanding of this mother's Jewish cultural and religious needs could have made her experience in hospital far less stressful.

References

Cohen, S. and Kahn-Harris, K. (2004) *Beyond Belonging: The Jewish Identities of Moderately Engaged British Jews.* London: UJIA.

Hoffman, L.A. (2002) *The Journey Home: Discovering the Deep Spiritual Wisdom of the Jewish Tradition.* Boston: Beacon Press.

Office for National Statistics (2001) Census. www.statistics.gov.uk/cci/nugget.asp?id = 954.

The Reform Synagogues of Great Britain (1985) *Forms of Prayer for Jewish Worship, Volume III, Prayers for the High Holydays.* London: The Reform Synagogues of Great Britain.

Tournier, P. (1957) *The Meaning of Persons.* New York and Evanston: Harper and Row.

Wallace, D. (2004) 'Spiritual Aspects of Dementia.' In S. Curran and J.P. Wattis (eds) *Practical Management of Dementia: A Multi-profession Approach.* Oxford and San Francisco: Radcliffe Medical Press, pp.207–218.

Further reading

Cooper, H. (ed.) (1988) *Soul Searching: Studies in Judaism and Psychotherapy.* London: SCM Press.

Jewish Hospital Chaplaincy Services, *Caring for a Jewish Patient,* Rabbi Martin van den Bergh (ed.), Senior Hospital Chaplain, Visitation Committee, www.jvisit.org.uk/hospital/caring-medical.htm.

Jewish Medical Ethics, www.jewishvirtuallibrary.org/jsource/Judaism/medtoc.html.

CHAPTER 8

THE INDIVIDUAL VERSUS THE FAMILY: AN ISLAMIC AND TRADITIONAL SOCIETIES PERSPECTIVE

Ahmed Okasha

Introduction

Six thousand years ago, Ancient Egyptians had healing temples where psyche and soma were one unity and patients were treated by both medication and healing through their mystical and spiritual beliefs. Egyptians were the first to worship one god and to believe in the afterworld without any prophets, which led James Breasted (1934) to write his book *The Dawn of Conscience*. From pharaonic times to Christianity to Islam, both Shiah and Sunni Egyptians always believed in the influence of spiritual healing and that the person united with the family is the basis for any treatment.

The separate functions of religious practice and healing were performed by a single individual in most world cultures. Only with the explosive growth of scientific knowledge in the twentieth century have the roles of religious and medical healers become separate.

We should be aware that all heavenly religions, whether Judaism, Christianity or Islam, and Eastern philosophies such as Hinduism, Buddhism, Confucianism and Taoism, advocate medicine for the person and that together with medicines, spiritual healing is an important issue. The emphasis of all these religions and their spirituality focuses not on the person but on the role of the person in relation to God and the family.

The Koran is divided into 114 chapters or *surahs*, whose main purpose is to proclaim God's omnipotence and mercy and man's total dependence on Him. Islam brought vast changes to the moral and social order of Arabia and established a specific system in which faith, politics and society were joined in the areas of social justice, special-interest groups, the status of women, race relations and the conduct of war. Mohamed taught respect for the natural world order, which allowed Muslims to approach science much earlier than Christians.

These directives became known as 'the medicine of the Prophet'. The Prophet stressed that 'for every disease there is a cause', which strongly persuaded followers to seek treatment. He understood psychological factors in disease, as indicated by his saying, 'He who is overcome by worries will have a sick body.' Muslim theologians believed that the Prophet advocated combining medicine with divine healing and physical treatment with psychological treatment, but with an emphasis on the family and community rather than the individual.

Medicine of the person in Islamic and traditional societies that are family oriented more than individually oriented will probably be more applicable if compatible with Islamic spirituality. The boundaries between the person and the family are so blurred that the person cannot perceive himself as an independent self or as having a separate existence from his family. This may explain the non-comprehension of the West for the implementation of democracy in other regions in the world. When these people go for election, they vote for the family or tribe and not for any plans or strategies for future development. They take their pride, achievement and sacrifice from belonging to the family. To illustrate how the person dissolves into the matrix of the family – however unacceptable it may appear – a child may be brought up until the age of 21 years for one purpose: the vendetta for the killing of his father or cousin, etc. His mother and siblings may take pride in sacrificing their son for the honour of the family although they know that he will be punishable by law and can be hanged according to Egyptian law.

This reveals the unification of the concept of the family and the person and how the person cherishes the loyalty, identification and fusion with his family. Medicine of the person as an integral part of the family and society has been practised in this region for a long time.

Impact of culture on the individual and family

Culture draws upon rich traditions of human thought and practice. An increased awareness of the impact of culture on individual and family reactions in contemporary societies has both positive and negative aspects. From a positive point of view, cultural belief systems may provide understandable explanations for traumatic life events or provide meaning for an individual or a group. From a negative point of view, any cultural fundamentalism, regardless of belief system, can be damaging not only to individual mental health and social adjustment but also to peaceful coexistence among cultures.

Throughout history, many authors have tried to describe the personality of whole nations, emphasizing certain behaviours and lifestyles that they believe to be representative of the 'national character' of particular nations. Among those authors who concerned themselves with the study of Arab/Islamic cultures was Ibn-Khaldun (1981) who is considered the real founder of the science of sociology.

Since Arab culture is very heterogeneous, with characteristics that vary from one community to another, the validity of a generalized concept like a unified 'national character' can easily be called into doubt. The current trend adopted by anthropologists and social psychologists is to avoid using terms like 'national', 'ethnic' or 'racial'. Kardiner *et al.* (1983) developed the concept of a 'basic personality type' that is shared by a group of people in a particular culture. They declared that the concept does not correspond to the total personality of the individual but rather to the projective systems or the value-attitude systems that are basic to the individual's personality configurations. Thus the same basic personality type may be reflected in many different personality configurations.

The following table highlights the main differences between traditional and Western societies. We understand that these generalizations do not apply to each and every individual and that each of those cultural dimensions are complex and multifactorial, yet we believe that it may still be useful in demonstrating the nucleus of the characteristics from which the different variations can be derived.

Cognitive style

The sociopolitical and economic systems and the child-rearing practices in Arab and other traditional cultures are completely different from those of Western cultures.

Al-Jabry (1986) summarized his opinion on the technique of the Arab mind in his book *The Structure of the Arab Mind*. He stressed that he what he meant by the 'Arab mind' was the total of principles and rules

Table 8.1 Main differences between traditional versus Western societies

Traditional society	Western society
Family and group oriented	Individual oriented
Extended family (not so geographical as before, but conceptual)	Nuclear family
Status determined by age and position in the family, care of elderly	Status achieved by own efforts
Relationship between kin obligatory	Determined by individual choice
Arranged marriage with an element of choice dependent on interfamilial relationship	Choice of marital partner, determined by interpersonal relationship
Extensive knowledge of distant relatives	Restricted only to close relatives
Decision-making dependent on the family	Autonomy of individual
Locus of control external	Locus of control internal
Respect and holiness of the decision of the elderly	Autonomous decision
Deference is God's will	Self-determined
Individual can be replaced. The family should continue and the pride is in the family tie	The individual is irreplaceable, self-pride
Pride in family care for the disadvantaged	Community care for the disadvantaged
Dependence on God in health and disease, attribution of illness and recovery to God's will	Self-determined

that Arab Islamic culture provides for those belonging to it as a base for acquiring knowledge and hence imposing it as a 'cognitive style'. He reported that the Arab mind is structured basically through dealing with the text in a literal sense, so that it deals more with words than with concepts. Similarly, Chaleby *et al.* (1999) believes that the developing Arab culture may still be functioning at a pre-operational stage and therefore Arabs prefer to deal with concrete rather than abstract formulations. That could explain the tendency of many Arab families to interact using concrete supportive and cognitive techniques rather than more abstract insight-oriented and non-directive techniques.

Language

Language as the main cultural instrument of communication creates meanings in a special way. For Arabs spirituality and religion are at the heart of creating meanings and purpose of living and also of the commandments concerning interpersonal relationships, which represent specific values and expectations. A Muslim's day is organized by regular rituals, each of which entail a remembrance of God and a verbal ritual that accompanies this remembrance; a fact that indicates the belief that man's destiny and fate are in the hands of a supernatural force beyond one's control except through personal obedience. Here it may be worth drawing the attention of the reader to the fact that the miracle of the Koran is essentially in its language. The multiple meanings and ways of expression associated with one event or subject reflect a richness, but also an evasiveness, of the language.

The overwhelming sense of belonging to a wider social structure and the widespread, dare we say, rejection of individuality is reflected in the use of 'we' while actually meaning 'I'. A common paraphrase used by Muslims upon saying the word 'I' is to follow it with an excuse: 'God protect me from the uttering of I'.

Spirituality and religion

Although spirituality and religion are often used interchangeably, religion contains so many unrelated variables that it cannot be considered a one-dimensional concept (Okasha 1999). Islam organizes Arab society. It is involved in every aspect of daily life. It is the source of moral values, legislation, and it shapes all aspects of social interactions, marriage and raising children. The positive effect of religion and faith cannot be ignored. People who believe in the hereafter can adapt more successfully to stress. Islamic rituals like group praying and fasting foster group identity and belonging. Islam stresses clearly that individuals are responsible for their actions but at the same time it acknowledges their limitations. Islamic rituals like scheduled praying and washing before praying aid in sublimating unacceptable desires and wishes. The notion of sin, which is deeply rooted in Western cultures, corresponds with the notion of shame as a driving force for behaviour in Arabic Islamic culture. Yet interestingly forgiveness is an important value in Islamic teachings.

However, religion is also what interpreters say it is. The interpretation of Islam has over centuries witnessed various orientations, at times leading society into progress and challenge of oppression, and at others being itself the tool of oppression. In the former role Islamic interpretations tend to highlight the role of an individual in creating his or her world, the individual responsibility for right and wrong, the ability of one's mind to differentiate between right and wrong, and the lack of intermediaries between God and His creations. In times of defeat and backwardness, exactly the reverse is stressed. The 'father', whether in the family, the mosque or the state, is the authority to be obeyed blindly, for it is he who will bear the consequences of the behaviours of individuals. Blind obedience becomes a virtue and using one's mind for questioning and exploration becomes unfavourable, sometimes amounting to sin.

Social and family systems

Contrary to Western cultures, Arab culture is strongly patriarchal. Patriarchal cultures tend to be group-oriented rather than individually orientated. Consequently the relationship between the individual and the family and society at large is one of interdependence rather than independence. The concept of autonomy in Western cultures is not applicable in Arab culture since it cannot be achieved without alienation from society.

While autonomy is considered a milestone of social growth and maturation in individually oriented societies, in traditional societies it is viewed as a wish to 'break free' from the rules of the family/clan/tribe and so on, and it is therefore frequently frowned upon.

Education at school and home is instructional and relies on giving advice and information, based on a parent–child or a teacher–student model. This model is replicated elsewhere, for example in religious institutions. Challenging that relationship breaches barriers of respect.

The 'father' in the family assumes the parent or the teacher position, being active, directive and judging. He may use him- or herself as a model for values and information that are not to be challenged. Heads of state may be referred to as family elder and hence are entitled to the same level of respect that a family member is entitled to, a dynamic which constitutes the basis for several dictatorships in the region.

A democratic parent is not one who provides space for independent choice and determination of lifestyle and patterns for his family, but one who is actively involved in establishing goals and offers a variety of transference reinforcements and responses to encourage the 'son' to achieve them. The conclusions and statements of the 'parent', judged subjectively, are taken as instructions to be followed. Family expectations of an individual are not only the guideline to behaviour but also the terms of reference against which one measures one's success or failure.

Individuality versus affiliation

In Eastern cultures, social integration is emphasized more than autonomy; that is, the family, not the individual, is the unit of society. Dependence is more natural and infirmity is socially acceptable and sometimes respected in these cultures. When affiliation is more important than achievement, how one appears to others becomes vital, and shame, rather than guilt, becomes a driving force.

The collectivity of the community is valued rather than the individuality of its members. Decisions are made not at an individual level but on a familial, tribal or communal level, in the best perceived collective interest.

The family structure is characterized by affiliated behaviour at the expense of differentiating behaviour. Also, child rearing is oriented towards accommodation, conformity, interdependence and affection versus individuation, intellectualization, independence and compartmentalization.

Dependence versus independence

Dependence in Arab and Islamic culture is both accepted and necessary. Their basic structure regards women as dependent on men (regardless of the claimed or declared discourse), the younger as dependent on the older and the masses as dependent on the governor. These are some overt modes of dependence. Many other implicit modes are working as strongly as the overt ones, and perhaps more so. For instance, parents are dependent on their children (especially when children are considered, usually unconsciously, as an investment).

A father–son dialectic relation under the umbrella of dependence on God is the basic relation judging most Arab Islamic parent–child relationships. This mode of relating and growth has been suggested by

Rakhawy (2000) to show how Arab Islamic culture differs basically along the march of growth. If this concept is proven and relatively accepted, it is likely to replace, at least partly, the famous Oedipal mode of relating that is claimed to be universal. In the parent–child dialectic, the parent–child conflict is established through shared dependence on a third common partner (God).

Along with variable degrees of dependence, individuals usually expect to have definite answers to their questions as well as definite instructions to follow. This is usually complied with, especially if dependence is accepted overtly by both parties.

It is culturally assumed that the 'father' is able to understand more profoundly and comprehensively than the 'son', regardless of their respective age. This includes the son's suffering, the causative factors, the whole situation, the son's needs and occasionally his future.

Understanding does not necessitate declaration or explanation. Nonverbal communication sometimes works in this respect better than declared agreement. It is related to 'the need to be seen' without being split or condemned or judged upon. It includes holistic perception, tolerance of ambiguity and the ability to postpone or even to avoid authoritative or moralistic judgement. This ability to understand the dependents silently and to let them lie 'in brackets' for an adequate time, with the least interference or judgement, is an indication of the wisdom of the elderly. No overt confrontation is made, but the judgement is felt and accepted.

Decision-making

In traditional societies, people tend to have an external locus of control and all events are considered to be God's will. Islam centers on the idea of a person's obligation or duties rather than on any rights he may have. One widely quoted verse from the Koran clearly states that man was created to worship God only. Against that background, autonomy and decision-making acquire a complex nature, trying to reconcile these duties with the requirements imposed by life.

In traditional cultures, individual concerns are dealt with as family matters. How to approach them is dependent not on what the patient wants him- or herself but on the estimation, need, or wish of the extended family. The individuals themselves may wish at times not to be burdened with the extra responsibility of making decisions that may determine the patterns of the rest of their lives. The concept of shared responsibility is central in traditional cultures, where most people would not like to be responsible for the outcomes of decisions made on their own (Okasha 2000).

Family expressed emotions

Considering that expressed emotion is a global index of particular emotions, attitudes and behaviours expressed by relatives about a family member, and that culture can be defined as a generalized coherent context of shared symbols and meanings that individuals create and recreate in their daily interactions, psychological anthropologists have shown that emotions can no longer properly be considered a private, intrapsychic or psychobiological phenomenon (Kleinman and Good 1984).

Traditionally in expressed emotion research, a certain number of criticisms has been used to separate patients' families into the two groups of low and high expressed emotion. Further analysis of the relationship between criticism and the occurrence of relapse into depression at various cut-off points of criticism showed that cut-off points between three and eight were significantly associated with relapse. The best prediction point came from dividing the groups at seven criticisms, the point at which the relative risk was highest (RR = 20.4). Thus, patients exposed to seven or more critical comments were 20 times more prone to relapse than those exposed to fewer than seven comments.

The relapse rate of 56 per cent in an Egyptian sample echoes relapse rates found in Western studies of depressive relapse and expressed emotion, for example 53 per cent (Vaughn and Leff 1976) and 51 per cent (Leff 1989) in two British studies, and 58 per cent in a US study (Milkowitz et al 1988). Married male patients had a higher relapse rate than female patients and were exposed to a significantly higher level of criticism as compared to female patients. This was attributed to several factors. Women in Arab Islamic cultures are exposed from childhood to various degrees of criticism and their gender tends to have inferior self-perception as a result. Their behaviour is continuously under scrutiny, either for social or traditional reasons. The occurrence of critical comments in the context of depression is therefore not necessarily perceived as a response to the illness, but rather a continuation of a normal process. This is in contrast to the attitude of the family towards its male members, where criticism or comments are made sparingly and with great care, so as not to injure the male 'dignity'. Criticism in the context of depression would be in stark contrast to the pre-morbid attitude of the family towards its male members. Another reason could be the social expectations from a male as the breadwinner for the family. An impaired social functioning would in this case cause much disturbance to the stability of the family and is therefore less tolerated. A third possible factor could be that in contrast to schizophrenia, depression is perceived more as a state of weakness and laziness than an illness (Okasha *et al.* 1994).

The finding that bipolar patients tolerated higher levels of criticism was rather unexpected. It appears, however to be in accordance with Okasha's (1988) view that outcome for the two types of depression differs. Perhaps some bipolar patients with existing hypomanic predispositions use humour as a coping device or buffer for criticism and thus dilute its potentially harmful effects. Further studies using larger samples are advisable to verify the relation of gender, type of depression and emotional expression.

It seems reasonable to postulate that cultural differences may explain why Egyptian patients relapse at higher rates of criticism than Western patients. We think that the level of 'domestic' criticism in the Egyptian culture in general could be higher than in English or North American homes. This interpretation is shared by Okasha (1988) and Akabawi (1990) who view high emotional expression as a kind of common social trait in Egyptian families. Hefny (1990) argues that criticism may sometimes actually be a sign of care and interest in Egyptian enmeshed families, a view shared by El-Islam (1979). Thus, it seems rational that there may be a higher level of 'usual' or 'benign' culturally accepted criticism in Egyptian families. El-Islam (1982) found that extended families in an Arab culture were more tolerant of eccentric behaviour and temporary withdrawal than were nuclear families. Those families encouraged more social activity without over-taxing the patient's social resources. Such behaviour is similar to low emotional expression responses to the patient's problem. Reactions like these by the extended family would not only produce a less stressful environment for the patient, but would model low emotional expression behaviour for members of a nuclear family. Consequently a substantially higher level of criticism, compared to Western samples, is needed to show its effect in the relapse of depressed patients.

Unfortunately, our expectation about the utility of perceived criticism as a predictor of relapse failed. This is unfortunate because training in the Camberwell Family Interview and emotional expression ratings is time-consuming and sometimes not feasible. Fortunately, however, there are promising data concerning the utility of the Five Minute Speech Sample as a brief screening device for measuring emotional expression (Malla *et al.* 1991). More work is needed in a cross-cultural perspective to know whether this more expedient method can be adopted as an established instrument.

Gender

Gender is a very complex issue in Arabic Islamic culture. Attitudes and opinions vary greatly from one Arabic society to another. The level of a person's education and social class along with exposure to Western values shape those attitudes and opinions.

There is a common but erroneous belief that traditions and social norms in Arabic cultures are derived from the religious teachings of Islam. Prohibition of sexual freedom and the extreme punishment for it are examples of an Islamic tradition that treats both males and females equally. That is to say, extramarital sex is just as prohibited for males as for females. Cultural traditions, however, do not frown on the extramarital sex of males, while considering the same action committed by female to deserve no less than death. This double standard is the core dynamic for many issues of gender discrimination. Wives have to put up with their husband's infidelity, since it is not considered grounds for protest. Unmarried girls are subject to abuse by young men who court them under the guise of love and intention to marry, only to leave them when they are no longer of interest to them. The common advice given by clergy to men with marital difficulties is, 'You may find yourself another wife'; the same adviser will tell a troubled and abused wife, 'Be patient, and God will reward you for it'. The less privileged status of women is also reflected in the bias of the services provided and the attitude of the medical profession, as will be discussed later.

It is one of the basic assumptions of Arabic and Islamic cultures that the man has the major responsibilities for making important decisions. Decisions like getting married have to be endorsed by the father; getting a divorce is a husband's prerogative. A woman cannot even go to work or school without the approval of her father or husband. Giving away vital personal and life-detrimental decisions to another person puts Arab women in a passive observant position to events happening to them and their person. In one of Chaleby's studies (1985), conducted on 270 patients, he found that women relate their psychiatric symptoms to the stresses in life significantly more than men do. He concluded that the position of being a passive observer to painful events is similar in many ways to the learned helplessness model described as one of the dynamics of depression.

Statistics covering the psychiatric services in Saudi Arabia showed that the numbers of women attending psychiatric clinics are lower than those of men. These statistics were derived from many sources, in different centres; almost all have attributed this finding to the fact that a woman cannot seek help of any kind for herself independently. She has to be driven to the hospital or a clinic. She therefore will not do so when she feels that her privacy is an issue. With psychotic conditions a woman will often not be treated until her psychosis becomes an embarrassment to her family, or at least too obvious to be ignored. Women are significantly over-represented in general practice clinics, because it is easier for the woman to ask her male guardian to take her to see a physician for a physical complaint than an emotional one. Somatization is consequently reported to be more prevalent in females.

Restricted freedom of movement has been reported to be a factor in child abuse and Munchausen's syndrome by proxy. Restriction of movement is also endorsed by law in several Arab countries where women are not allowed to be issued with passports or travel without prior permission of their guardian, father or husband. Even when she has their permission to have a passport, the husband or father still retains the right to stop her from travelling at the airport. This extends into the years of adulthood of a female, stressing her status as a second-class citizen. The stress induced by this restriction varies depending on the need to travel (being highest when travelling is necessary to increase family income for example) and the level of awareness (inducing greater sense of anxiety among women who are aware of the subordination that this entails) (Chaleby 1986).

In Arab culture a woman cannot choose to be independent even if she is able to do so. There is a simple rule stating that no woman is expected to live alone. A popular saying is that to be in a man's shadow is better than to be in the shadow of a wall. However, the sense of entrapment that results can be a source of many stresses contributing to the state of helplessness. A woman can be trapped in a marriage she does not accept, not only because the decision of divorce is a man's prerogative, but even if her husband is willing to comply with her wishes, if she is to escape from a dissatisfying relationship she has only one alternative and that is to live back in her father's house, or, if he is dead, with her brother, which can be worse than living with her husband in the first place. An unmarried woman is so uncomfortable in her single status that she might accept any offer of marriage just to be out of the house. That would especially be the case when she is facing a cruel father or a rejecting brother and sister-in-law. But even when this is not the case, a divorced Arab woman is stigmatized among her family and neighbours, and no matter what the reason for the divorce, she always has to live with the guilt that it was her fault she could not maintain the marriage (Chaleby 1988).

Chaleby (1999) studied the mechanism and nature of social and family interaction in Arab culture for many years. One of the important observations made was that the Arab individual is usually more concerned about the impression given to others than the one actually perceived by the individual him- or herself. This statement applies more to women. Furthermore, the woman is usually more concerned about her status with the man than about her own achievements. Many females will easily end a successful career for the sake of satisfying their husbands, or try to appear less intelligent to gain the approval of the man. The Arab woman is brought up to centre her individuality, self-perception and sense of identity around the presence of a man.

Conclusion

In conclusion, it remains to be highlighted that this individual–collective relationship does not go unrewarded. In exchange for the dependence and control imposed by a hierarchical family and societal structure, the individual does not only bear the responsibility of adhering to the norms of the collective, but also enjoys being its responsibility. Individuals in traditional societies go through a lot to 'belong' even if it means subverting some of the collective norms. In exchange, individuals enjoy the lack of anguish of being left on their own once they are in trouble, ill or old. Until now, and despite the strong waves of modernization that sweep the world, those values seem to hold. True, they might be maintained by those who benefit from them in terms of social status and the power that they grant. However it seems that less powerful beneficiaries are also not too anxious to change them.

Finally we should not overlook the fact that such 'social support' elements do not merely translate in the field of humanities. Social networks and social support have been shown to stimulate neurogenesis and increase connectivity among dendrites in the brain, especially in the hippocampus, which is responsible for coping strategies, adaptation to stress, social learning, memory and mood. Thus the differences in interpersonal relatedness and self-image, although socially expressed, may in fact also be an expression of a brain mechanism that is either affected by, or itself shapes the psychological need of people, or both.

References

Akabawi, A. (1990) Personal communication.

Al-Jabry, M.A. (1986) *The Structure of the Arab Mind.* Beirut: Markas Drassat Al-Wahda Al-Arabeia.

Breasted, J.H. (1934) *The Dawn of Conscience.* New York: Scribner's.

Chaleby, K. (1985) 'Women in polygamous marriages in an inpatient psychiatric service in Kuwait.' *J Nerv Ment Dis 173,* 56–58.

Chaleby, K. (1986) 'Psychosocial stresses and psychiatric disorders in an outpatient population in Saudi Arabia.' *Acta Psychiatr Scand 73,* 147–151.

Chaleby, K. (1988) 'Traditional Arabian marriages and mental health - study in an outpatient group of Saudis.' *Acta Psychiatr Scand 77,* 139–142.

Chaleby, K. and Racy, J. (1999) 'Psychotherapy with Arab patients toward a culturally orientated technique.' In Chaleby's and Racy's *Psychotherapy with the Arab Patient.* Tuscan, AZ: McLaughlin/QSOV.

El-Islam. M.F. (1979) 'A better outlook for Schizophrenics living in extended families.' *Br J Psychiatry 145,* 343–347.

El-Islam, M.F. (1982) 'Arabic cultural psychiatry.' *Transcult Psychiatr Res Rev 19,* 5–24.

Hefny, K. (1990) Personal communication.

Ibn-Khaldun, A.M. (1981) *Muqaddimah Ibn-Khaldun.* Beirut: Dar al-Qalam.

Kardiner, A., Linton, R., DuBois, E. and West, J. (1980) In H.I. Kaplan, A.M. Freedman and B.J. Sadock *Comprehensive Textbook of Psychiatry,* 3rd edn. Baltimore/London: Williams & Wilkins.

Kleinman, A and Good, B (eds) (1984) *Culture and Depression: Studies in the Anthropology and Cross-cultural Psychiatry of Affect and Disorder.* Berkeley: University of California Press.

Leff, J. (1989) 'Controversial issues and growing points in research on relatives' expressed emotions.' *Int J Soc Psychiatry 35,* 133–145.

Malla, A.K., Kazarian, S.S., Barnes, S. and Cole, J.D. (1991) 'Validation of the five minute speech sample in measuring expressed emotion.' *Can J Psychiatry 36,* 297–299.

Milkowitz, D.J., Goldstein, M.J., Nuechterlein, K.H., Snyder, K.S. and Doane, J.A. (1988) 'Expressed emotion, affective style, lithium compliance and relapse in recent onset mania.' *Psychopharmacol Bull 22,* 628–632.

Okasha, A. (1988) *Clinical Psychiatry.* Cairo: Anglo Egyptian Bookshop.

Okasha, A. (1999) *Religion and Mental Health at the Turn of the Century.* Plenary Events, XI World Congress of Psychiatry, Hamburg, Germany, 6–12 August.

Okasha, A. (2000) 'The impact of Arab culture on psychiatric ethics.' In A. Okasha, J. Arboleda Florez and N. Sartorius (eds) *Ethics, Culture and Psychiatry: An International Perspective.* Washington, DC: American Psychiatric Press.

Okasha, A., El Akabawi, A., Wilson, A., Youssef, I. and Seif El Dawla, A. (1994) 'Expressed emotion, perceived criticism, and relapse in depression: A replication in an Egyptian community.' *Am J Psychiatry 151,* 151–157.

Rakhawy, Y. (2000) 'Psychotherapy in Egypt (An Overview).' In A. Okasha and M. Maj (eds) *Images of Psychiatry, An Arab Perspective.* Cairo: Scientific Book House.

Vaughn, G.E. and Leff, J.P. (1976) 'The influence of family and social factors on the course of psychiatric illness: A comparison of schizophrenia and depressed neurotic patients.' *Br J Psychiatry 129,* 124–137.

CHAPTER 9

HINDU AND AYURVEDIC UNDERSTANDINGS OF THE PERSON

Dinesh Bhugra

Introduction

The concept of the self is at the root of our existence and identity and so-cial and psychological functioning. The phenomenological approach came into its own in the late nineteenth and early twentieth centuries in order to understand the self and the psychopathology of the self. This ap-proach differed from behaviourism and psychoanalysis in that for phe-nomenology the basic subject matter of psychology is the psychological experience of the individual at any particular moment in time. It is the in-dividual's direct perception of the external world and how it is experi-enced and responded to which constitutes the subject matter of psychology. The relationship between the subjective world, the objective world and culture and society therefore leads to a new way of looking at the individual.

Although Paul Tournier was aware of other faith traditions, his un-derstanding of personhood, and of medicine of the person, was derived from within a Christian 'Western' perspective as well as from develop-mental psychology. Other ways of looking at the significance of the per-son include the Hindu and Ayurvedic traditions described in this chapter, which emphasize the links to the absolute and to the spiritual world.

In this chapter I shall define the self-concept and link it with Hindu and Ayurvedic traditions.

Self-concept

Self-concept is and remains an unequivocally subjective phenomenon (a key component of the individual's phenomenal field), and yet it is also a social product originating from social interaction and being constantly influenced by social experience. What we see of ourselves is determined by how we see ourselves and also how we see others seeing us. Whatever decisions we make are predicated on some implicit assumption of what we are like. Self-concept is the totality of the individual's thoughts and feelings with reference to themselves and can be characterized in terms of diverse dimensions, different regions, different planes, and so on (Rosenberg and Kaplan 1982).

Religion is one of the key aspects of an individual's cultural identity. Belonging to groups based on common beliefs is important, albeit these groups do not necessarily need to be entirely religious (see Table 9.1).

Table 9.1 Social identity

1. Social status	Sex
	Age
	Social class
2. Membership groups	Cultural identity
	Common beliefs, e.g. religion, sociopolitical, interests
3. Labels	Stealing: *Thief*
	Drinking: *Alcoholic*
4. Derived status	Ex-convict
	Emeritus Professor
	Alumnus
5. Types	Vague, e.g. geeks
6. Personal identity	Deepest thoughts, feelings and wishes

The individual may well choose not to identify with the group and status of social category (by rejecting the group), but may still be recognized as a member, especially if he or she is identified as a member by others.

Within social identity, social expectation and personal worth too play a role in the individual's response. Concepts of traits implicit in roles play a major role in identification of self-concepts and social responses. Griffith and Bility (1996) suggest that for any religious beliefs and thinking to emerge, social and cultural factors have to be taken into account. The beliefs can be seen as arising and developing in three similar stages, perhaps parallel to the evolution of the groups: the predisposing, empowering and operational phases.

Littlewood (1996) argues that conditions in which personal psychopathology can be communicated are at an individual disease and illness level, and people and time define these. Social, political, economic and cultural factors too play a role, thereby making it possible for the individuals to either fight with these factors or come to a mutually beneficial arrangement. The beliefs of individuals, if extreme, may have an almost delusional flavour and fervour. Both religion and psychiatry are interested in changes of heart, attitude or behaviour, yet it is likely that their responses will differ markedly. This allows the individuals to respond in different ways as well. Evans (1985) argues that arousal states within an individual due to behavioural changes may also be more suggestible, making it likely that individuals with extreme beliefs are looking for further increased arousal in newer religious movements or extremist religions.

Concepts of the self

It is important to differentiate between self-concept and constituents of the self. The former as defined above is the concept an individual holds of himself or herself and how others perceive that self, whereas the latter is more to do with a structure of the self and its interaction with external factors. Identifying one's values and self-conception is not to be confused with ideal self or ego ideal.

The self-concept is most frequently described sociologically as naming the roles that are prominent in it (see Table 9.2).

Such derived categories allow the researcher and clinician alike to place the individual in a specific context, which allows the individual's self-concept to change along with the specific context. The systematic sense of self includes a sense of moral worth, self-determination, unity and competence (see Table 9.3) and these four senses are correlated with system functioning, which allows the individual to achieve certain goals including integration within the self and with the society (Table 9.4).

Table 9.2 Derived categories (after Gordon 1982)

A. Ascribed characteristics	Sex
	Age
	Racial heritage
	Name
	Religious categories
B. Roles and memberships	Kinship roles
	Occupation
	Social status
	Territoriality
	Membership of a group
C. Abstract identification	Existential
	Abstract, e.g. human
	Ideological and belief, e.g. liberal
D. Interests and activities	Judgements
	Intellectual concerns
	Artistic activities
E. Material references	Possessions
	Physical self
F. Systemic senses of self	Cultural and social identity
G. Personal characteristics	E.g. personality, how to act
H. External meanings	Judgements imputed to others, e.g. popular
	Situational references, e.g. late, early

Self-concept and self-esteem

Kaplan (1975) argues that even though the acquisition of the self-esteem motive is normal, it is relative frequency of positive and negative self-descriptions and characteristics of responses to self-devaluing situations and histories that influence maintenance of self-esteem.

It can be argued that the relationship between the individuals, their self-concept and their self-esteem is further complicated by the fact that a perception of focus of control also tends to play a role, along with prejudices as perceived by black and minority ethnic groups, for example.

Table 9.3 Systematic senses of self (after Gordon 1982)

Senses	Characteristics
Moral worth	Self-respecting, sinner, bad, good, honest (preponderantly attributive)
Self-determination	Ambitions, wanting to get ahead, self-starter (almost always attributive)
Unity	In harmony, mixed up, ambivalent (predominantly attributive)
Competence	Intelligent, talented, creative, skilful (primarily attributive)

Whether a cultural deprivation is worse than social/economic deprivation in determining the individual's self-esteem and self-concept needs to be studied further.

Table 9.4 Relationship of self and system functions

System function	Corresponding sense of self
Adaptation	Sense of competence
Goal attainment	Sense of self-determination
Integration	Sense of unity
Pattern-maintenance	Sense of moral worth

Rosenberg and Pearlin (1978) demonstrated from schools in Chicago and Baltimore that for adults the self-concept often included others from different socioeconomic status, whereas for children by virtue of their school attendance such a differential did not exist. Rosenberg (1979) suggests that the following three key points are identified:

1. That the self-concept components are of unequal centrality to the individual's concerns and are hierarchically organized in a system of self-values.

2. That the self-concept can be viewed at both the specific and global levels.

3.   That the self-concept may consist primarily of a social exterior or of a psychological interior.

Psychological centrality of the self-concept cannot be denied. As Tournier (1957) highlights, the way in which 'we' personage is inextricably bound up with the person in spite of the fact that we always tend to think of the role we play as different from what we are in reality. Thus concept of the self and its relationship with reality are at the core of individuals' functioning. However, its relationship with *maya* or (illusion) in Hinduism becomes of greater interest.

Another aspect of the self-concept, which is of interest in the present discussion is the 'desired' self-concept. Rosenberg (1979) goes on to describe this as our picture of what we wish to be like. The desired self consists of three components – the idealized image, the committed image and the moral image. Idealized image is driven, insatiable, frustrated and indiscriminate. Any preoccupation with this image will lead to intense strain, increased sensitivity to criticism and extreme vulnerability. Horney (1945) argues that ultimately all this leads to self-hatred and self-contempt.

Motivations and self-concept

Self-concept motives are related to self-seeking and self-preservation (James 1890) or the maintenance or enhancement of the self (Snugg and Combs 1949). Two separate motives of self-esteem and self-consistency are incorporated in the self-concept. Self-consistency incorporates protection of the self, self-preservation, maintenance of the self and self-concept stability. It refers to the motive to act accordingly with the self-concept.

One of the interesting observations reported in the literature (Fitch 1970) suggest that persons are motivated to perceive events in a way that enhances low self-esteem and is also consistent with chronic low self-esteem. Interestingly those with low self-esteem may adamantly refuse to accept information that will improve their self-esteem. Epstein (1973) argues that those with low self-esteem may retain low self-esteem in order to protect their self-esteem. Thus people with low self-esteem may set their aspirations to a level that allows them not to over-reach and fail.

Religious beliefs and self-concept

By studying children in ten high schools in New York State, Rosenberg (1962) hypothesized that dissonant context may well have a differential effect on individuals from different religious groups. He found that the experience of living in a dissonant religious context has certain psychic consequences for the individual exposed to it.

In every case students who had been raised in a dissonant social context were more likely than those who had been raised in a consonant or mixed religious environment to manifest symptoms of psychic or emotional disturbance.

Bhugra *et al.* (1999) found that Asian women who held less traditional and more 'modern' attitudes were more likely to attempt deliberate self-harm because there was a clearer conflict with the community.

Hindu tradition

Hinduism is a way of life, a philosophy as well as a religion that influences social systems, functioning at social and individual levels, and an intricate pattern of living that feeds into the self-concept of individuals. Hindu tradition talks of the self either to reject its ontological status or to assimilate it in a theological and metaphysical construct, but there appears to be a rejection of the egocentric self (Bharati 1985).

Hinduism is not a school of philosophy in the traditional sense but its six components of philosophy deal with analysis, dualism (but dualism as between man and nature), materialistic philosophy (a rational and naturalistic system of metaphysics), number-circulation or reason (thoroughgoing rational philosophy), atheistic doctrine and philosophy of salvation. These schools grew individually and gradually. The ground of the universe – that the only reality is the spirit and the individual soul (*atman*) – is identical with the reality of the spirit. This reality is often described in Sanskrit by the term *saccidananda* meaning absolute consciousness (*cit*) and absolute bliss (*ananda*).

According to the texts, the relationship of the self to the eternal unchanging reality, *Brahma*, is seen as essentially unreal and the world as an illusion – the maya. The world is neither real nor unreal and its appearance is based on the reality of the ultimate spirit – *Brahman* (see Morris 1994 for further discussion).

Salvation is achieved through the practical realization (not merely the theoretical awareness) of the identity, the oneness of the self (*atman*) with the absolute (*Brahman*).

Within Hinduism what the schools have in common is the salvation involving the detachment of the individual from the phenomenal world. The dualism as noted earlier is not between mind and body but between nature and man, or between spirit and phenomenal world.

Hindu self

From the Hindu perspective the soul is encased in three bodies – the physical body, the subtle body (sound, touch, colour, taste, smell) and the subtle bhutas (which consists of the mind (*manas*), intellect (*buddhi*) and the vital energy (*pranas*). Thus all Hindu notions about the mind, cognition and the entire psychological aspects of life are seen in philosophical terms as material conceptions as part of the phenomenal world of change and *karma* (Morris 1994). The individual has layers (*kosa*) where the self is formed of body, then the senses, the mind, the intellect and finely the *atman* (which equals *brahman*), the ubiquitous absolute that has no form and no matter (Bharati 1985). Thus the two selves – phenomenal or material self and an inner self – is associated with spirit, being formless, immutable and absolute.

The realization of the true self is therefore implicit in detachment from the phenomenal world of becoming, not only from desires and material attachments, but also from the flux of psychic life itself. The three secular goals of life are *karma*, *artha* and *dharma*. *Karma* means desire or pleasure, and the hedonistic aspects of life are important in the context of Hindu culture as evidenced by erotic sculptures, sexual monographs, plays, music and other art forms. As Morris (1994) points out, some scholars tend to underplay the hedonistic aspects and focus more on puritanism. *Artha* refers to the wealth and possession of material gains using honest means for worldly success including pursuit of social, political and material goals. The third goal of *dharma* is living life according to the sacred or moral law. Roughly translated as duty, sacred order, essential nature of a being and right conduct, it is often confused with religion. It also means the upholding of custom and law. *Dharma*, argues Morris (1994) also postulates a divinely sanctioned social order. The similarities to Plato's castes of guardians, military auxiliaries and artisans are worth bearing in mind.

Although the broad division of Hindu society into four castes was prevalent the subdivisions were much more complex and the caste system linked to the theory of *karma*. The highest value of life's aim is to reach *moksha* – the liberation or release from the cycle of rebirth.

Not only are there four castes and four goals in life there are four stages in one's life, starting from the state of *brahmcharya* (celibacy) for the first quarter of one's life, followed by a stage of *grahastha* (which is equivalent to being a householder or getting married and having children).

The third stage is *vanaprastha* (where the individual starts to do social things and fulfil social obligations) and the last stage is *sanyasa* (i.e. giving up worldly goods and the renunciation of family ties). Four paths to salvation are those of knowledge, action, devotion or philosophy.

Dumont (1970) identifies two conceptions of individuals among Hindus – the individual as the empirical agent and rational being, and as the normative subject of institution. Individual identity is achieved by repudiating all ties which bind the person to the caste system and the world. In an ordinary everyday context the Hindu identity is linked to kinship and caste membership and the interpersonal identity is social rather than metaphysical. The empirical self among Hindus is weak and ephemeral but the real self is spiritual; the notion of 'I' is pure consciousness divided between social and spiritual self.

Ayurveda

Ayurveda (literally, the science of life) has several textual sources starting from the Vedic period. *Atharvaveda* (the last of the four Vedas) has mentioned illnesses and their remedies in a magico-religious context but the beginnings of an empirical–rational medicine were clearly present. Charaka and Susruta were the two physicians who produced an early codification of ancient Indian medicine. Psychiatry in ancient Indian texts was reviewed by Bhugra (1992). A more detailed treatment of the basic concepts of Ayurveda in relation to mental health and therapeutics can be found in Frawley (1998); Ramachandra Rao (1990); and Dash (1989).

Ayu (life) is the combined state of body, senses, mind and soul. The body is made up of the five *mahabhutas* (proto-elements, namely earth, air, fire, water and space). In contrast to the body–mind dualism in Western psychology, *manas* (mind) in Ayurveda is regarded as *ubhayatmaka*, an organ that mediates between body and soul, as it is primarily a creation of space. As it is active throughout the body its seat of control lies between *siras* (head) and *talu* (hard palate). It has three *gunas* (qualities): *Satva, Rajas* and *Tamas*. These three qualities lead to different behavioural patterns.

These are the pathogens of the mind just as *vata, pitta* and *kapha* are the pathogenic factors in the body and these provoke intense emotions and cause conditions like *udvega* (anxiety) and *vishada* (depression). They are called *gunas* in Sanskrit, meaning 'what binds', because wrongly understood they keep us in bondage to the external world. The three *gunas* are one of the prime themes of Ayurvedic thought and influence *doshas* (humours) just as the latter can affect the former. In fact, derangements of all the four entities (body, senses, mind, soul) interact and even if one of them is deranged, the remaining three are also affected. Mind is described as a surface part of consciousness through which the external world is seen and interpreted. This outer mind is called *manas* in Sanskrit, which means the 'instrument of thinking'. It is the sixth sense organ used for ideas and emotions. It is also the sixth motor organ, ruling over the other five, and expressing ideas and emotions.

The state of *manas* is understood by its functions like *indriyanigraha* (perception and motor control), *manonigraha* (mental control), *ooha* (guess/imagination) and *vichara* (thought). Ramu, Venkataram and Janakiramaiah (1988) analysed the *manovikaras* (mental disorders) with reference to *udvega* (anxiety) and *vishada* (depression). These two conditions are prototypic examples of the etiological class of disorders known as *manasika* (psychological). In contrast are the *saririka* (physical) group of disorders. Those disorders in which both body and mind are aetiologically involved are grouped as *ubhayatmaka* (psychosomatic/somatopsychic).

There are five kinds of *unmada* (psychosis), namely *vata, pitta, kapha, sannipata* (all three *doshas* are vitiated) and exogenous. The four kinds of psychosis excluding the exogenous are caused by imbalance of *doshas* manifesting themselves rapidly in the following circumstances:

1. when an individual is timid

2. when he is mentally agitated

3. when the *doshas* in the body are aggravated and vitiated

4. after partaking of unwholesome or unclean food

5. when the body is greatly emaciated

6. when suffering from any other diseases

7.   when the mind is constantly afflicted by passion, hatred, anger, greed, excitement, fear, an attachment, exertion, anxiety and grief.

Its premonitory symptoms are desire for inflicting injury upon pious and innocent beings, irritability, peevishness, apathy, impairment of *ojas* (primal vigour), nightmares and lack of lustre and strength. The symptoms are extraordinary strength, energy, ability, prowess, grasping power and retention of knowledge. In *unmada*, fully fledged disease symptoms manifest immediately after the premonitory symptoms. In this respect, *unmada* is different from other diseases, in all of which the actual manifestation of the disease occurs a long time after the premonitory symptoms develop. The self in the Hindu context therefore is not isolated self but is seen as and functions as a contextual matter.

The general line of treatment, taking into account the *doshic* balance and the *satwa* of the individual besides disease-specific procedures in certain conditions, is extensively used by Ayurvedic physicians in treating various mental disorders (in modern terminology, anxiety disorders, depressions, psychoses, alcoholic syndromes and somatoform disorders).

Yoga

Yoga is the other major Indian tradition that is relevant to understanding medicine and psychiatry. It aims at 'the calming of the operations of consciousness' according to Patanjali's *Yogasutras*. The practice of yoga, it is therefore claimed, can reverse all psychological problems.

A detailed description of various procedures under each variety of yoga was given by Iyengar (1976).

Medical applications of yoga used predominantly *asanas*, *pranayama* and meditation. Meditation refers to 'a family of techniques which have in common a conscious attempt to focus attention in a non-analytical way and an attempt not to dwell in discursive, ruminating thoughts' (Shapiro 1982). It is the process of attending to the objects of one's awareness more than the particular contents of awareness, which is important. Meditation procedure can be broadly one of two types: concentration meditation or awareness meditation. Here the self is seen as being controlled by one's own actions.

Rosenberg (1979) argues that self-concept is the totality of the individual's thoughts and feelings having references to himself (*sic*) as an object and it is the picture of the self. By highlighting the concepts of social identity as a key part of the self-concept he argues that social identity includes gender, race, nationality, religion, family status, legal status, name, etc. He divides social identity into social status, membership groups, labels, derived status, types and personal identity.

All these components encourage the individual to cope with stresses and strains and with each component in place, the concept of self allows the individual to function at their best.

Hypothetical model: Self-concept and its relationship with external factors such as political, social, economic and cultural factors can lead to a hypothetical model as illustrated in Figure 9.1.

Environmental/   Internal factors
external factors

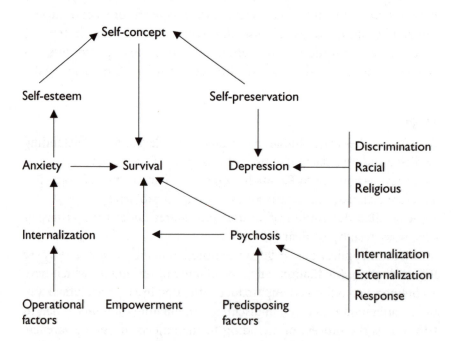

Figure 9.1 Hypothetical model

In summary, Ayurveda and yoga influence the Hindu view of the self and can play a significant role in the management of psychiatric disorders. The application of specific procedures to different disorders merits examination. Biological effects during these therapies need to be identified and their role in mediating therapeutic effect defined. It is also important to learn from their holistic ideas and lifestyle philosophies in order to more effectively prevent disease and promote health. It would be useful to develop a databank on the therapeutic applications of Ayurveda and yoga in mental health.

Learning points

- Hinduism is a way of life and a philosophy.
- The concept of self is kinship based.
- Ayurvedic approaches are holistic.
- Patients may use pluralistic approaches.

References

Bharati, A. (1985) 'The self in Hindu thought and action.' In A.J. Marsella (ed) *Culture and Self: Asian and Western Perspectives.* London: Tavistock.

Bhugra, D. (1992) 'Psychiatry in ancient Indian texts: a review.' *History of Psychiatry 3,* 167–186.

Bhugra, D., Bhui, K., Desai, M., Singh, J. and Baldwin, D. (1999) 'The Asian cultural identity schedule: an investigation of culture and deliberate self-harm.' *International Journal of Methods in Psychiatric Research 8,* 212–218.

Dash, V.B. (1989) *Fundamentals of Ayurvedic Medicine.* Delhi: Konark.

Dumont, L. (1970) *Honio Heirarchious: The Caste System and its Implication.* London: Weidenfield and Nicholson.

Epstein, S. (1973) 'The self-concept revisited.' *American Psychologist 28,* 404–416.

Evans, P. (1985) 'The Process of Religious Conversion and Psychological Change.' In E. Chiu (ed) *Pyschiatry and Religion.* Conference proceedings, St Vincent's Hospital, Melbourne.

Fitch, G. (1970) 'Effects of self-esteem, perceived performance and choice on causal attributions.' *Journal of Personality and Social Psychology 16,* 311–315.

Frawley, D. (1998) *Ayurveda and the Mind: The Healing of Consciousness.* Delhi: Motilal Banarsidass Publishers.

Griffith, E.E.H. and Bility, K. (1996) 'Psychosocial factors and the genesis of new African American religious groups.' In D. Bhugra (ed) *Psychiatry and Religion.* London: Routledge.

Gordon, M.M. *Assimilation in American Life.* New York: Oxford University Press.

Horney, K. (1945) *Our Inner Conflicts.* New York: Norton.

Iyengar, B.K.S. (1976) *Light on Yoga: Yoga Dipika.* London: Unwin.

James, H. (1890) *The Principles of Psychology.* Reprint 1950. New York: Dover.

Kaplan, H. (1975) 'Prevalence of the self-esteem motive.' In H. Kaplan (ed) *Self-attitudes and Deviant Behaviour.* Pacific Palisades, CA: Goodyear.

Littlewood, R. (1996) 'Psychopathology, Embodiment and Religious Innovations: An Historical Instance.' In D. Bhugra (ed) *Psychiatry and Religion.* London: Routledge.

Morris, B (1994) *Anthropology of the Self: The Individual in Cultural Perspective.* London: Pluto.

Ramachandra Rao (1990) *Mental Health in Ayurveda.* Bangalore: National Institute of Mental Health and Neurosciences.

Ramu, M.G., Venkataram, B.S. and Janakiramaiah, N. (1988) 'Manovikaras with special reference to Udvega (Anxiety) and Vishada (Depression).' *NIMHANS Journal, 6,* 1, 41–46.

Rosenberg, M. (1962) 'The dissonant religious context and emotional disturbance.' *American Journal of Sociology 68,* 1–10.

Rosenberg, M. (1979) *Conceiving the Self.* Malabar, FA: Kreiger Publishing.

Rosenberg, M. and Kaplan, H.B. (eds) (1982) *Social Psychology of the Self-Concept.* Arlington Heights, IL: Harlan Davidson.

Rosenberg, M. and Pearlin, L. (1978) 'Social class and self-esteem among children and adults.' *American Journal of Sociology 84,* 53–77.

Shapiro, D.H. (1982) 'Clinical and physiological comparison of meditation and other self-control strategies.' *American Journal of Psychiatry 139,* 267–274.

Snugg, D. and Combs, A. (1949) *Individual Behaviour: A New Frame of Reference for Psychology.* New York: Harper.

Tournier, P. (1957) *The Meaning of Persons.* Reprinted 1972. New York: Harper and Row.

PART 3

MEDICINE OF THE PERSON IN CONTEMPORARY PRACTICE

CHAPTER 10

SPIRITUALITY AND MENTAL HEALTH: PRACTICAL PROPOSALS FOR ACTION

Peter Gilbert

It is 24 April. Is the date important? Perhaps, as a student of history, I am sometimes obsessed by dates and events; as someone said, 'History is just one…event after another'. Former Prime Minister Harold Macmillan, when asked what politics was about, replied: 'Events, dear boy, events'.

So, it is Sunday 24 April and I am driving my car to take part in the Stratford-upon-Avon Half Marathon; running, and the wellbeing that derives from it, being a major part of my spirituality (of which more later). Turning on the car radio I expected to hear *The Archers*, a soap opera I have been addicted to for many years, and which tends to cover many of the contemporary angsts and preoccupations of contemporary life: for instance the schemes of the arch materialists Lillian and Matt Crawford; the issues of identity for Emma, Will and Ed, as we wonder which brother is little George's father; and Tom's struggle for a more rounded approach to his humanity, rather than just building up his business empire.

In fact, *The Archers* had been broadcast much earlier in the day, and BBC Radio 4 was featuring the inauguration of Pope Benedict XVI. The fact that the British media had covered the illness, death and funeral mass of Pope John Paul II with such assiduity and solemnity – and indeed that both the Royal Wedding and the announcement of the date of the British general election had been delayed – was extraordinary, considering the Reformation-sourced nature of the British Constitution (see Kettle 2005b). Were the British media fascinated with the character of an individual with demonstrable spiritual strength and integrity, whether one agreed with his policy pronouncements or not, or was there also some, perhaps reluctant, attraction to an enduring institution in a rapidly changing and somewhat anomic world (see Bauman 2000)?

Martin Kettle, one of *The Guardian*'s leader writers, and someone who was a couple of years ahead of me at Balliol – a noted intellect with a radical turn of mind – found himself writing another article on Pope John Paul II, where his attention was drawn 'repeatedly – and sometimes unwillingly –…back to the most public private ordeal that many of us have witnessed' (Kettle 2005a). Kettle pointed out that:

> John Paul is also doing more than fight for his own life. He seems to be using his position and fame to make a statement about all our lives…he is saying that his suffering is universal. But he is saying, above all, that all lives are valuable, and that he is entitled to live his life to the very end, however hard it may be. (Kettle 2005a, p.20)

In many ways, the drama of the death of one spiritual leader, and the elevation and inauguration of another, has been a colourful depiction of some of the current discourse of meaning and identity in the tewnty-first century. John Paul II's successor, Cardinal Joseph Ratzinger, was seen by many as the late Pope's 'enforcer', but in his sermon at the funeral mass of his mentor, Ratzinger made a statement that encapsulates much of our current dilemma:

> There is the desert of poverty, the desert of hunger and thirst, the desert of abandonment, of loneliness, of destroyed love. There is the desert of God's darkness, the emptiness of souls no longer aware of their dignity or the goal of human life. The external deserts in the world are growing, because the internal deserts have become so vast…the Church as a whole and all her pastors, like Christ, must set out to lead people out of the desert, toward the place of life, toward friendship with the Son of God, toward the One who gives us life and life in abundance. (Joseph Ratzinger, 24 April, 2005)

This short, mystical statement incorporates many of the questions that haunt us: does contemporary life give or deny meaning? (Frankl 1959); whether the search for a greater celebration of individuality should be tempered by a consideration of community and uniqueness (see Appiah 2005; Rolheiser 1998; Sacks 2002); is the value of life being undermined? (Fromm 1976; Vardy, 2003); is the pursuit of happiness making us actually happy? (Layard, 2005 and Hutchinson et al 2002; Putnam

2000); whether there is a transcendent being, or whether transcendence is a condition within ourselves; and whether institutional religion is a path to a better life (or merely a rope line), or are the institutional imperatives always going to swamp the humanitarian ones?

Enduring questions that come out of a dialogue with individuals and groups are:

- Can individual and individualized spirituality reach out in a wider circle of community(ies), or would such an extension to others contaminate or dilute the very essence of meaning that starts with the existential person?

- Can organizations, in an era of rampant performance measures, move from the transactional to the transformational and so make human services actually human! (see Gilbert 2004, and 2005b).

As Bernard Moss puts it in one recent contributions to this subject:

> The issues of religion and spirituality take us to the very heart of what it means to be human and to be living together in society. For me, there are profound connections between religion, spirituality and social justice; between the 'tap root' of compassion and the human rights of those who are marginalised, oppressed and victimised. They are of deep significance…and deserve to be taken seriously by anyone who works professionally in the human services. (Moss 2005, p.1–2)

These of course are by no means new questions; they are as old as time. Recent research on cave paintings in western Europe has demonstrated that the paintings were not intended as we usually intend artistic endeavours, namely to be shown off to other human beings; they were depicted in inaccessible places, presumably as an offering to some form of transcendence.

The ancients in their writings speak of the essential congruence of body, heart and spirit. As Plato put it:

> As you ought not to attempt to cure the eyes without the head, or the head without the body, so neither ought you to attempt to cure the body without the soul…for the part can never be well unless the whole is well. (Quoted in Ross 1997, p.3)

As well as ancient philosophies, the major religions also talk about a defining fire or spirit within the human entity which is essential to its wellbeing and development. The Hebrew word *ru'ach* means both breath and spirit, as does the Latin *spiritus*. Hindus believe that in each person there dwells the breath of the Divine – *Atman*; and Muslims speak of the necessity of looking to the health of the spirit, which has its domain in the *qualb*, the human heart (see Sheikh and Gatrad 2000; NIMHE/MHF 2003).

As well as looking at the wholeness of the individual, the world religions have also considered the totality of the physical world (or created world if you believe in a Creator). There have been contradictions here, especially as some Christian thinkers have been as dualistic in their conceptions as some of the rationalists they have criticized.

Muhammad Salim Khan, writing in his text on Islamic medicine, states that:

> The whole edifice of Islam is based on an understanding of *Tawhid* – a primordial concept of the oneness and unity of all creation... Unity as a method perceives the cosmos as a dynamic, integrated and purposeful whole...every aspect of Islamic thought and action rotates around the doctrine of unity, which Islam seeks to realise in a human being in his (*sic*) inward and outward life. (Khan 1986, pp.24–25)

Throughout the Renaissance and Enlightenment the debate raged, and we see it played out as much in novels as anywhere else, as in George Eliot's *Middlemarch* (1872), where the Chair of the local hospital, Mr Bulstrode, and the Dr Lydgate, are found engaged in conversation:

> 'I am aware' he (Bulstrode) said, 'that the peculiar bias of medical ability is towards material means. Nevertheless, Mr Lydgate, I hope we shall not vary in sentiment... You recognize, I hope, the existence of spiritual interests in your patients?'
>
> 'Certainly I do. But these words are apt to cover different meanings to different minds.' (Eliot 1964 [1872], p.124)

Up to the present day we see in books and films, and the public response to them, a thirst for a discourse around good and evil; religion and spirituality; life and death; the spirit and the material – in works by such as J.R.R. Tolkien, Philip Pullman, Ursula LeGuin and J.K. Rowling – and, as the fictional Dr Lydgate points out, spirituality has many meanings!

The Australian David Tacey (Tacey 2004), who is very sceptical about institutional religion, as he is indeed about purely individualized spirituality, shakes the tree of secularism when he declares that:

> But the ideals of secularism, however well-intended, are inadequate for life, since our lives are not rational and we are hugely implicated in the reality of the sacred, whether or not this is acknowledged. (Tacey 2004, p.12)

Quantum physicists are now challenging the materialist nature of the human brain and the human cosmos. Physicist Danah Zohar and psychiatrist Ian Marshall postulate from the new sciences that:

> There is a third kind of thinking of which the brain is capable, and hence a third intelligence connected inherently to meaning... It flies in the face of twentieth century cognitive science, which sees mind essentially as a computation machine. (Zohar and Marshall 2000, pp.86–87)

The economist Richard Layard, a government adviser on economic practice, asks the pertinent question as to why, at a time of economic prosperity 'we are not happier than we are. Why is there so much anxiety and depression?' (Layard 2005, p.26). John Swinton, suggests that humankind is 'hard-wired for spirituality' (Swinton 2001). In the field of industry and commerce commentators are focusing on whether organizations are able and willing to provide the meaningfulness that so many seek (Howard and Welbourn 2004; Alford and Naughton 2001; Holbeche and Springett 2004). Dr Andrew Powell, as founder member of the Royal College of Psychiatry's Special Interest Group on Spirituality and Psychiatry, has spoken of the dissonance between the search by people who use mental health services for a spiritual aspect of their struggle against the more reductionist training of medical practitioners (see Croydon Mind 2005).

Survivors of mental distress, such as Sue Holt, describe in their poetry the desire to talk of the transcendent and the constraints placed upon them:

> I was excited; today was the Lord's birthday
> and I was going home for dinner
> I masked my emotions
> otherwise they would keep me
> I had to behave myself today

no talking of God
and of his plans for me
and the future of the world
my family came for me
eventually. Waiting is such pain.

(From 'Year 2000 on a Section 3', Holt 2003, pp.98–99,
reproduced with permission)

My own path to leading the National Institute for Mental Health in England (NIMHE) Project on Spirituality and Mental Health came from a crisis of meaning. While we are familiar with high staff turnover in the public sector, partly due to stress and dissatisfaction with an increasingly mechanistic ethos, one of the strange, secret scandals of modern Britain is the sausage machine that chews up and spits out senior managers in the public sector (usually in the high-risk areas of social services and NHS trusts), at an alarming rate. A crisis occurs, usually due to deep-seated structural (e.g. political or financial) problems and, instead of having the moral courage to face the issues head-on, those in charge go for the instinctive reaction of changing the pilot at the helm. In the developing world we would be shocked, but in Britain it is a drama played out constantly, though usually behind closed doors and only rarely hitting the headlines. I came into a newly constituted local authority in 1997, as Director of Social Services. It was an authority with a long history of financial crises, poor relations with the NHS and other partners, and at least one vital childcare indicator at the lowest level in England and Wales. A 7 per cent cut in an already non-viable budget saw an inevitable crisis several years later, and the perhaps predictable knee-jerk reaction.

Faced with early retirement after 31 years of public service (the army, then social work and social services), in a state of high activity and anxiety, as I strove, on two hours sleep a night, to keep the ship off the rocks, followed by a deep depression, the abiding image I have is of the time in my early twenties when I went climbing with the Italian Alpine Regiment and came off a mountain ledge a couple of thousand feet high. Dangling helplessly, watching the rocks through my splayed feet, and totally reliant on other people to help me back to the safety of another ledge, was exactly how the depression felt like.

Like many people who find themselves leading public services, I probably have an exaggerated sense of responsibility and accountability. Although those with a detailed knowledge of the politics, personnel and finances of the authority reassured me that it was not my fault, I inevitably felt I was responsible, and voices from childhood, when academic attainment was a struggle for me, came back to haunt me – another common experience of people experiencing a crisis of mental health, meaning and identity. It is still an abiding disappointment in those I worked for, that nobody from the authority contacted me whilst I was off sick with depression for six months, or subsequently. If I had been found hanging from Worcester Bridge, no doubt there would been suitable expressions of shock and horror. I have been fortunate to re-build my career, and on the national stage, whereas many of my colleagues have simply disappeared, at great loss to the common good. It has been of some wry amusement to me to note how 'resurrection' is always profoundly embarrassing to those who have erected the crucifix or scaffold! Political juntas always prefer the 'disappeared' to remain firmly disappeared – the 'dead' to remain buried. As T.S Eliot wrote, how perilous it is when corpses are exhumed (*The Waste Land* 1922).

While much of the six months remains a blur, I can vividly remember what helped. I was very fortunate to have a GP who was both technically sound, human in her approach, and who gave me a measure of control. She advised sleeping pills and anti-depressants. Like many people, perhaps, I was reluctant to take the anti-depressants, perhaps because I didn't want to admit I was ill. When I did take them I found they worked rapidly, and with minimal side-effects (although I know that this is not the experience of many). Perhaps what helped most, however, was that my GP was undisguisedly angry at the state I was in when I came to her from working in an ostensibly caring agency. Other aspects that helped me were a friend who had been through a similar experience, who, like me, was a runner, and both listened and gave me good advice, while we drank endless cups of tea or pounded the Worcester canal paths. Another friend, from a minority background, and therefore no stranger to discrimination and scapegoating, was particularly good at absorbing my pain, distress and anger. Most people feel very uncomfortable at the expression of strong feelings, because they perceive them as a threat. This friend was able both to empathize, absorb and also be angry on my behalf.

For many years, I had found the Benedictine Abbey at Worth in Sussex (see BBC2, *The Monastery*, May 2005; *The Monastery Revisited*, June 2006; and Jamison 2006) a place of both sanctuary and development; somewhere to get back in touch with a natural rhythm of life which was often missing from the world I found around me. *In extremis* I found the

Abbot and his community exemplars of the Benedictine ethos of hospitality, and rediscovered the Rule of St Benedict as a model of 'servant leadership', which was a sound corrective to the mechanistic model I had recently experienced (see Gilbert and Jolly 2004). Another facet of my struggle to regain wellness and move into recovery (see Allott, Loganathion and Fulford 2002) was running. For me, running has aspects of the physical, the spiritual, and maybe even of the religious (Gilbert 2005c; Jamison 2006). Not only does running release endorphins, a natural response of the body to cope with the physical effort, which leads to a 'high' (see Mental Health Foundation 2005), there are benefits in terms of feeling closer to nature and the physical world; stimulating a sense of beauty; communing with others – either conversing, or simply being with them, but in one's own space (mental, physical and emotional); providing a sense of inspiration, hope and achievement; creating a sense of solidarity and teamwork with other runners; and giving a sense of meaning and identity (Coyte forthcoming).

As the depression lifted and I felt able to work again, though 'full' recovery took about 18 months, I was fortunate to be asked to take on some work by people I respected – a very valuing experience after an episode of devaluation. One of those people was Professor Anthony Sheehan, at that time the Lead for the Department of Health on Mental Health, and the Chief Executive of NIMHE, then in the process of formation. Professor Sheehan invited me to be NIMHE's Lead for Social Care, and it was a very inspiriting time to work for somebody with vision, passion and integrity. One of the core group meetings to set up NIMHE (which was launched in the summer of 2002) took place only a couple of weeks after the traumatic and iconic events of 11 September 2001, when Al-Qaida operatives attacked what they saw as the totems of Western capitalism: the World Trade Centre, the White House and the Pentagon. Although many papers branded them as 'mediaevalists', in fact, as one commentator pointed out, the majority of the terrorists were disillusioned technocrats. Anthony Sheehan recognized that, although NIMHE was already working on policies and practice around the experience of people from black and minority ethnic groups, the issues of individual spirituality and faith, and in the light of 9/11, specific issues around those faiths feeling under threat (Geaves 2005), would need specific attention, and he set up a specific project to focus on this.

Work on black and minority ethnic issues has grown apace in mental health, from the publication of *Inside, Outside* in March 2003 (NIMHE), through to the consultation framework document of October 2003 (Department of Health (DoH)), to the action plan of February 2005 (DoH), which contains also the Government's response to the independent inquiry into the death of David Bennett. Of course spirituality is not purely related to ethnicity, though it is a major connecting issue; the essential link is one of humanity, starkly put by Dr Joanna Bennett, speaking at the inquiry on her brother's death in care, when she pleaded for services to 'just get the humanity right!' (quoted in Gilbert 2005b, p.11).

The aim of the NIMHE Spirituality and Mental Health Project, which commenced essentially in the autumn of 2001, is to:

> Collate current thinking on the importance of Spirituality in Mental Health on an individual and group basis, to evaluate the role of faith communities in the field of mental health and to develop and promote good practice in whole persons approaches. (NIMHE/The Mental Health Foundation 2003, p.5)

Inspiring Hope sets out both the objectives of the project and the outcomes expected. It is perhaps worth quoting that the first outcome is for 'a recognition and practical application of the importance of the spiritual dimension in people's lives' (p.9), and the first three objectives are to:

1. Chart what is known and who is doing what in terms of:

   - The role of spirituality in mental health
   - The role of religion in mental health
   - The role of faith communities in mental health

   via a research and literary search and work, to identify sites of good practice in mental health services (including primary care, the voluntary sector and user-led initiatives) and in faith communities.

2. Build coalitions of individuals and groups who are willing and able to combat stigma, discrimination and exclusion, and to promote the value of positive mental health as a vital element in the health of the nation.

3. Develop and create linkages with the other NIMHE programmes and with other networks and initiatives in this sphere.
   (NIMHE/The Mental Health Foundation 2003, p.5)

In November 2003 the project was re-launched at the project's first national conference, *Breath of Life.*

It is vitally important that this work is not seen as yet another example of performance management. It needs to *breathe*, and work on a partnership and collaborative basis. To this effect constructive links have been built with the existing national Spirituality and Mental Health Forum (previously hosted by Mentality, and now hosted on a rotating basis by different groups, currently the Jewish Association for the Mentally Ill (JAMI); the Three Faiths Forum, and specific faith groups and their social policy and practice manifestations. With the Church of England holding a particular place in national life, and often being a bedrock of chaplaincy services, there is a strong relationship with the Church of England's Adviser on Home Affairs at Church House; and recently the project, and members of the Department of Health and Church of England advisory team met with Dr Rowan Williams, Archbishop of Canterbury, for a full discussion of mental health issues in general and the project in particular. One of the outcomes was the offer by the Archbishop of one of his Inter-Faith Forum meetings to take the project further.

Because it is vital that the project is not seen as representing organized religion but is helping in the promotion of the whole persons and whole systems approach generally, with an accent on the individual expression of the spiritual dimension, the project has created strong links with other NIMHE programmes and, in some senses, because of its emphasis on essential humanity, it could be seen to underpin much of the work that is going on. Some of these programmes are Race Equality, Workforce, Acute Care, Values, Recovery and Social Inclusion. Service users and carers often complain that their spiritual needs, or matters of religious observation, are simply not attended to by professionals, so that influencing professional and other forms of education and training are an essential part of the programme. The Royal College of Psychiatrists has had a special interest group for a number of years, and spirituality featured at the Royal College's annual conference in Edinburgh in June 2005. The British Psychological Association also has a section devoted to holistic care and one on trans-personal approaches.

As a social worker, it has been disappointing to see the under-development of this area in social work education and training, perhaps because of the in some senses quite justified suspicion of institutional religion at the time of social work's growth and development in the 1970s. The former Education Council for Social Work, CCETSW, criticized the lack of attention to this area and called it 'ever the invisible presence in modern social work' (Patel, Naik and Humphries 1997); Professor Phyllida Parsloe expressed concern that social workers 'seldom raise spiritual questions and I suspect that they sometimes make it difficult for clients to raise them' (quoted in Moss 2005, p.4); and Gilligan and others' recent research demonstrates that though there is a growing sympathy among social workers for considering the spiritual dimension, there are issues of confidence, which appear to restrict the profession, putting a great deal of stress on 'whole persons and whole systems' approaches from wholeheartedly embracing this issue (Gilligan 2003; Gilligan and Furness 2006).

One of the ways of taking this forward has been the preparation of a report for the new social work regulatory and educational organization, the General Social Care Council (GSCC) in a paper dated 5 June 2004, and the recent conference, hosted by Staffordshire University and the Higher Education Academy's Social Policy and Social Work Group, on 28 April 2005.

Work has been pulled together for the project by a small team, Project Lead Peter Gilbert from NIMHE and Project Co-ordinator Vicky Nicholls from the Mental Health Foundation (2003–2005). The Project Lead and Project Co-ordinator met bi-monthly with two interlocking groups: one comprising the eight reps from the eight NIMHE regional centres (since April 2005, part of the Care Services Improvement Partnership), followed by a meeting with the steering group, which consists of users, carers, academics, professionals, representatives of faiths, etc. The work of the project is informed by a standing group of users/survivors and the discourse that comes from the conferences, seminars, workshops, etc., which are held across the country.

Some of the current work includes collating examples of 'developing practice' (we deliberately did not use the phrase 'good practice' because of its loaded nature), which is financed by a Section 64 grant from the Department of Health. In the spring of 2005, a series of pilot sites were also set up, two to three in each region, which are designed to consider, and move forward, issues around spirituality and inspiriting organizations concerned with the mental health of the population. Most of these pilot sites are Partnership Trusts, but some are an interesting amalgam of different organizations in one geographical area. The Project will ascertain where the organization is currently; how humane and spiritual approaches are recognized, supported and celebrated; the assessment of spiritual and religious needs, and the care practice in a broad sense; recognizing and responding to an individual's spiritual needs, and also their religious needs; chaplaincy services; partnership approaches to faith communities, and also to community groups with a spiritual dimension; recognizing the spiritual and religious needs of staff; education and training processes; assisting faith communities in their understanding of mental health, and how they can work appropriately with services; published materials; and issues such as diet, space, interpreters, etc.

All the pilot sites are very much served by volunteers who recognize this as an important issue and want to share practice. A symposium drawing together all the pilots took place at the University of Lincoln in May 2006. The work will then be written up and helped to promote further developments; it is hoped that the pilot sites will continue for a number of years, as these are natural regenerative processes.

In terms of work with faith communities, this is an ongoing process, and network organizations such as the Inter-Faith Network have been most helpful. It has also been important to work across the major voluntary groups in this area such as Mind, Rethink, the Sainsbury Centre for Mental Health, Mentality, the Mental Health Foundation, Age Concern etc, as they, and many others, have all produced specific literature around spirituality and faith. Following the Archbishop of Canterbury's interfaith seminar, it is planned to have a symposium at Staffordshire University, with the nine faiths which are consulted by government departments in official consultation exercises, and the Humanist Society, where there are formal presentations on each institution's views on both mental wellbeing and mental illness, and how their theology and pastoral care interact. It is thought that this would be a ground-breaking approach, and would begin to build a sense of shared interest and shared concern across the different faith communities and with secular spirituality.

The knowledge base on this whole area is expanding enormously. One PhD student remarked to the author recently that when he started his doctorate research there were a limited number of sources. 'Now,' he complained in jest, 'I wish we could have a moratorium on the subject, so I can finish my doctorate in peace!' Some universities, such as Aberdeen and Staffordshire, have set up specific centres for spirituality, with strong support from the very top of the organization; in the case of Staffordshire, from Vice Chancellor Professor Christine King. To build on this growing momentum, a research forum was initiated during 2005 on a UK-wide basis, to start drawing together the knowledge base. Professor Bill

Fulford, NIMHE's Fellow on Values, is particularly concerned that the work on values and spirituality is closely linked, and national organizations on developing the knowledge-base, such as the Social Care Institute for Excellence (SCIE), have been very supportive. The spiritual approach demands that values and knowledge are held closely together; as Dr Samuel Johnson once put it: 'Integrity without knowledge is weak and useless, knowledge without integrity is dangerous and dreadful' (quoted in Gilbert 2005a).

In the twenty-first century, the era of post-modernism means that the 'grand narratives' of modernism, science and religion have been replaced by our own personal narratives, which both give us more power over our lives, but perhaps less solidarity with others. For many, the individual narrative has at last begun to be heard, and this is in some ways reinforced by Governmental policy around the choice agenda, and the need to hear the consumer voice. One of the worries, however, is that we all become 'mere consumers', individualized purely to become pawns and prey to global capitalism. As Zygmunt Bauman puts it in his text on *Liquid Modernity*:

> A cynical observer would say that freedom comes when it no longer matters. There is a nasty fly of impotence in the tasty ointment of freedom cooked in the cauldron of individualization; that impotence is felt to be all the more odious, discomforting and upsetting in view of the empowerment that freedom was expected to deliver. (2000, p.35)

Spirituality is clearly a facet of our individual humanity, linked to aspects of uniqueness, meaning, identity, purpose, relationships, a sense of the holy, and the spirit and fire which drives us (NIMHE/The Mental Health Foundation 2003; National Youth Agency 2005; Rolheiser 1998), but perhaps we should also be working towards creating communities of meaning, so that we are not simply adrift on a surging sea of change but are able to, if not put down anchors, at least arrange the sails and the crew so that we gain some solidarity sailing on the sea of life.

References

Alford, H. and Naughton, M. (2001) *Managing as if Faith Mattered.* Indiana: University of Notre Dame.

Allott, P. Loganathion, I. and Fulford, W.K.M. (2002) 'Discovering Hope for Recovery from a British Perspective.' *International Innovations in Community Health* (special issue). *Canadian Journal of Mental Health 21,* 3.

Appiah, K.A. (2005) *The Ethics of Identity.* New Jersey: Princeton University Press.

Bauman, Z. (2000) *Liquid Modernity.* Cambridge: Polity Press.

Coyte, M. (forthcoming) *Title to be confirmed.* London: Mental Health Foundation.

Coyte, M.E., Gilbert, P. and Nichols, V. (forthcoming) *Spirituality and Mental Health Care: Jewels for the Journey* (working title). London: Jessica Kingsley Publishers.

Croydon Mind (2005) *Hard To Believe.* DVD version. Croydon: Croydon Mind.

Department of Health (2003) *Delivering Race Equality: A Framework for Action.* Mental Health Services, Consultation Document. London: DoH.

Department of Health (2005) *Delivering Race Equality in Mental Health Care: An Action Plan for Reform Inside and Outside Services.* London: DoH.

Eliot, G. (1964 [1872]) *Middlemarch.* New York: Cygnet Classics.

Eliot, T.S. (1922) *The Waste Land.* London: Faber and Faber.

Frankl, V.E. (1959, first published 1946) *Man's Search for Meaning.* New York: Simon and Schuster.

Fromm, E. (1976) *To Have or to Be?* London: Johnathan Cape.

Geaves, R. (2005) *Aspects of Islam.* London: Darton, Longman and Todd.

Gilbert, P. (2004) 'It's Humanity, Stoopid!' Inaugural Professorial Lecture, published in Staffordshire University (2005). *Explorations.* Stafford: Staffordshire University.

Gilbert, P. (2005a) 'Spirituality and the Social Work Curriculum.' Presentation at *Spirituality, Religion and the Social Work Curriculum: The Neglected Dimension?* SWAP/Staffordshire University, 28 April.

Gilbert, P. (2005b) *Leadership: Being Effective and Remaining Human.* Lyme Regis: Russell House Publishing.

Gilbert, P. (2005c) 'Keep up your Spirits?' *Openmind.* September/October.

Gilbert, P. and Jolly, L. (2004) *Serving to Lead: St Benedict and Servant Leadership.* Sussex: Worth Abbey, July.

Gilligan, P.A. (2003) 'It isn't discussed: religion, belief and practice teaching: missing components of cultural competence in social work education.' *Journal of Practice Teaching in Health and Social Work 5,* 1, 75–95.

Gilligan, P.A. and Furness, S. (2006) 'The role of religion and spirituality in social work practice: views and experiences of social workers and students.' *British Journal of Social Work, 36,* 617–637.

Holbeche, L. and Springett, N. (2004) In *Search of Meaning in the Workplace.* Horsham: Roffey Park Institute

Holt, S. (2003) *Poems of Survival.* Brentwood: Chipmunka Publishing.

Howard, S and Welbourn, D. (2004) *The Spirit at Work Phenomenon.* London: Azure.

Hutchinson, F. Mellor, M. and Olser, W. (2002) *The Politics of Money.* London: Pluto Press.

Jamison, C. (2006) *Finding Sanctuary: Monastic Steps for Everyday Life.* London: Weidenfeld and Nicholson.

Kettle, M. (2005a) 'His Greatest Performance'. *The Guardian,* 26 March, p.17.

Kettle, M. (2005b) 'It's as if the Reformation had never happened.' *The Guardian*, 5 April, p.20.

Khan, M.S. (1986) *Islamic Medicine.* London: Routledge and Keegan Paul.

Layard, R. (2005) *Happiness: Lessons from a New Science.* London: Allen Lane.

Moss, B. (2005) *Religion and Spirituality.* Lyme Regis: Russell House Publishing.

National Youth Agency (2005) *Spirituality and Spiritual Development in Youth Work.* Leicester: NYA.

NIMHE (2003) *Inside, Outside: Improving Mental Health Services for Black and Minority Ethic Communities in England.* Leeds: NIMHE.

NIMHE/The Mental Health Foundation (Gilbert, P. and Nicholls, V.) (2003) *Inspiring Hope: Recognising the Importance of Spirituality in a Whole Person Approach to Mental Health.* Leeds: NIMHE/The Mental Health Foundation.

NIMHE (2005) *Up and Running: Exercise Therapy in the Treatment of Mild and Moderate Depression in Primary Care.* Leeds: NIMHE/The Mental Health Foundation.

Patel, N., Naik, D. and Humphries, B. (1997) *Visions of Reality: Religion and Ethnicity in Social Work.* London: CCETSW.

Putnam, R. (2000) *Bowling Alone: The Collapse and Revival of American Community.* New York: Simon and Schuster.

Rolheiser, R. (1998) *Seeking Spirituality.* London: Hodder and Stoughton.

Ross, L. (1997) *Nurses Perceptions of Spiritual Care.* Aldershot: Averbury.

Sacks, J. (2002) *The Dignity of Difference: How to Avoid the Clash of Civilisations.* London: Continuum.

Sheikh, A. and Gatrad, A.R. (2000) *Caring for Muslim Patients.* Oxford: Radcliffe Medical Press.

Swinton, J. (2001) *Spirituality in Mental Health Care: Redicovering a Forgotten Dimension.* London: Jessica Kingsley Publishers.

Tacey, D. (2004) *The Spirituality Revolution: The Emergence of Contemporary Spirituality.* Hove: Brunner-Routledge.

Vardy, E. (2003) *Being Human: Fulfilling Genetic and Spiritual Potential.* London: Darton, Longman and Todd.

Zohar, D. and Marshall, I. (2000) *SQ: Spiritual Intelligence, the Ultimate Intelligence.* London: Bloomsbury.

CHAPTER 11

BEYOND THE SOLITUDE FOR TWO: JUSTICE, THEOLOGY AND GENERAL PRACTICE

Thierry Collaud

Translated from French by Alister and Janet Cox

General medicine in tension between two traditions

In the last pages of his seminal book *Medicine of the Person* Paul Tournier tells the story of a patient tormented by important existential questions who had asked him to review them with him. The doctor suggests that they should spend three days together in the mountains. This is a story with an image of the doctor that has always fascinated and attracted me: an available person who is capable of extracting himself for a few days from daily preoccupations to devote himself to a patient. It is also the encounter that fascinated me, the complicity I imagined evolving between these two people in the course of the *therapy*. But although it attracted me as an ideal scenario, the situation always seemed to me completely unrealistic in the context of general medicine.

Unrealistic because it considers only one of the two faces of medical practice: this hypertrophied face-to-face encounter, in the isolation of the mountains, was totally divorced from the rest of the world, a point which is well made when Tournier tells how he had to explain to his ten-year-old son why he was going to leave him for some days. Now the various ways available for defining general medicine as well as its synonyms (family medicine, community medicine, medicine of the first resort) all make reference to the anchoring of this medical practice in the community. It is this anchoring that creates in general medicine a constant tension between relational and community aspects – one might say between singularity and plurality. The episode described above demonstrates this tension insofar as at one and the same time we find it appealing and yet unrealistic.

The danger lies in considering oneself obliged to choose between the two aspects in tension. In the context of medicine of the person it is most likely that we will favour the approach that sees it as an intense and rich encounter: the community side of our work will be understood only as the negative element, which is going to prevent us taking a patient to the mountains. Yet contrary to what one might expect, general medicine must integrate the two aspects, the personal and the communal. This integration is necessary for the simple reason that the two aspects are inseparable.

I shall argue that every relationship with others is surrounded and conditioned by multiple third parties. That is, there can never be something called a *private consultation* between patient and doctor if one understands by that a kind of *solitude for two*, with their links with the wider human community being temporarily suspended.

I believe that on the contrary it is only when we take these links seriously that we can enter into the real task of caring. I shall attempt to equate the notion of 'taking seriously' with that of justice, showing that this is in effect the relational harmony, the mutual respect, that one seeks to maintain between members of a community. We shall see that there are different ways of conceiving justice, and our preference will be for a wide definition that draws its inspiration (however paradoxical this may seem) from the theological tradition.

To refuse to take sides with one or other of the poles described above does not imply the disappearance of either of them (patient or community), but rather that they remain in a state of critical tension, neither being absorbed into the other. Each needs to be protected from the damage that would result from excessive exposure.

Face-to-face relations: the danger of the excluded third party

Michael Balint, whose influence on the doctor–patient relationship is universally recognized, entitled his world-famous book *The Doctor, his Patient and the Illness*. The big absentee in Balint's focus on the healer–healed couple is what might be called the *communal third party* – other people, all of them. Where are they? How important are they in this relationship? Are they intruders whom we should chase away in order to preserve the purity of the face-to-face relationship – or rather the forgotten element in this relationship, which it is absolutely necessary to reinstate so that dialogue acquires greater truth and depth? This question has inescapable relevance at a time when the excluded third party reappears in economic guise, knocking at the surgery door.

The face-to-face doctor–patient relationship has played a major role in the history of medical practice: the general assumption has been that the essence of what the doctor did for the patient is embodied in the privacy of the doctor–patient interaction. Current practice underlines the point: the privacy of the doctor's surgery, the closed door isolating him from the outside world – an isolation underpinned by the code of secrecy that surrounds what the two say to each other. When we speak about medicine of the person, we all too easily reinforce this interpretation by assuming that the main aspect of the healing relationship is the meeting between the person of the doctor and the person of the patient. A scenario that typifies Paul Tournier's practice is the prolongation of his conversation with the patient into the evening: they chat by the fireside in his own home. This reinforces the impression of a private space: the surrounding darkness, the fire providing light and warmth to the two protagonists. The image has emotional force – a solid one-to-one relationship constructed through withdrawal from the world.

I do not want to suggest that Paul Tournier's aim was to leave the world behind in the company of his patients, but rather that we all have within us a yearning for some warm and sympathetic relationship. It is not the relationship itself that invites criticism: we shall return to its importance later. The fault lies in the introverted aspect of the relationship as thus conceived, which not only ignores the rest of the world but totally excludes what I called the 'third party'; the others, all those not there in the surgery, not only those who are near and dear to the patient but every member of the community, whether local or far-flung. In this sense an internal requirement of every relationship can be said to be an openness to others: the risk otherwise is of an introverted duo, rigid and sterile.

The philosopher Emmanuel Levinas ably demonstrates that we can never entirely take in the person we meet as we would do an impersonal object (Levinas 1969). There will always be something in him that opens out towards the infinite beyond, not least the world of other people. It is this 'opening out' which prevents the relationship from closing in on itself in a 'complicity of privacy'. This view of things does not compromise the one-to-one relationship. On the contrary, it infinitely extends its scope: for the more I commit myself to the person in front of me, the more I recognize the need to go beyond the 'I–You' to the opening out to the wider world that this implies. 'The third party looks at me in the eyes of the Other' is Levinas' way of saying that the person in front of me can make me intimately aware of the presence of humanity, where the philosopher speaks of 'the epiphany of the face qua face opens humanity' or of 'the epiphany of the face inasmuch as it attests to the presence of the third party the whole of humanity, in the eyes that look at me' (Levinas 1969, p.213). We should think then not of a solitary one-to-one encounter in the privacy of the surgery but of something paradoxically different: the concept of a mass of folk clamouring to be let in.

To put it differently, the closed duo is impossible because each of us brings with us a multitude of 'third parties' who cannot be ignored. The patient is there before me with the life he has lived and with the life that opens up before him, with his beliefs, his values, his hopes and his fears. This is what constitutes his identity as a human being, his role within one or many scenarios, the relational spaces in which many others play their part. Repositioning the patient within this scenario, ensuring he does not cut himself off from his circle of acquaintance, this helps him take responsibility for his own recovery.

If the patient brings with him such a wealth of relationships, equally the doctor should not render himself inhuman by cutting himself off from the person he really is, becoming nothing but an 'expert' (a sort of super-computer) who gives the patient a choice between several therapeutic options (a false notion of autonomy). This may at present be the main danger he faces – that of suppressing his personality in order to fit into the mould of 'provider', satisfied with 'doing his job' in an impersonal way. It is on the contrary his own personal history and all the characters who people it, his beliefs and his values, his concepts of truth and falsity, right and wrong, which provide the background for his meeting with the patient on a person-to-person basis. This is a favourite theme of Paul Tournier, encapsulating his philosophy of 'medicine of the person'.

This analysis of the face-to-face relationship, in tension with the inevitable and necessary presence of the 'third party', shows up the fundamental ambivalence in any caring relationship. Being alongside, building a relationship, certainly implies a movement of withdrawal and retreat from the surrounding world (what happens strictly 'between us' is on a different level of intensity from that of other wider relationships), yet at the same time this retreat cannot be total insofar as my dialogue with another must take into account his 'role within the world'. One cannot therefore detach oneself totally from the world that clings to one's skin.

Serving the community: a threat to the personal dimension?

In a tradition that prizes the irreplaceable richness of the doctor–patient relationship we very often forget that the doctor is above all a carer. This means that he is not there in front of the patient on his personal initiative but because he has been put there in a sense by society. It is this society which trained him as a doctor and transmitted to him the knowledge which he possesses and applies, delegating to him society's caring function at the patient's side. We should not however forget that this caring function expresses itself in the attitude of a lot of different people and not simply the doctor. Even though for centuries he could believe that he was the uncontested master of the healing relationship, he is fortunately compelled nowadays to descend from so lofty a stance and recognize that 'taking care' is not his business alone but is basically a collective task.

He must also recognize that he is not the primary carer surrounded by a multitude of others but that he is one amongst others. Indeed what differentiates a doctor from a nurse or a chaplain is not the caring capacity, not the capacity for compassion – the capacity to join others in suffering and go together with them on a healing road. This caring aptitude is common to all of them and can be exercised by all. What differentiates health professionals consists only in the variety of technical skills. It is only on this technical and organizational level of care that the doctor can claim a certain hierarchical superiority over the other professions. At the level of pure caring capacity he remains one amongst equals.

When considering the caring function within the workings of a health care system and more widely of society at large, we must take into account the danger of depersonalization that is inherent in such a system. Granted that no personal interaction is possible without reference to the wider social background (what I have called the 'third party'): there is on the other hand the possibility of social interactions that lack all personal reference. What I mean is that human *action* can be transformed into a bare and inhuman *doing*, if care is not constantly taken to maintain interaction with others in the level of personal relations: we must not let them degenerate until people are treated as objects; see Buber 1987, who distinguishes these two kinds of relations, called by him 'I–Thou' and 'I-It'; see also the notion of human action described by Hannah Arendt in *The Human Condition* (1998 [1958]).

THE FASCINATING THIRD

The danger thus defined makes its appearance under different guises, both fascinating and repellent. Amongst the fascinating elements there is technical progress; the dream of a science where everything can be explained, foreseen, regimented; systems that know no limits. In the excitement of this and of a handful of successes, doctor and patient alike dream of guaranteed cures and the total eradication of disease. It is an alienating fascination that takes over, filling all their mental space and diverting them from a relationship where the acceptance of our mortality offers the possibility of journeying together through life and savouring its pleasures. Turning their backs on this and in the vain pursuit of life, they sacrifice (as the Roman poet put it) for the purpose of living the very things which make life worth living: '*et propter vitam vivendi perdere causas*' (Juvenal 1999 [exact date unknown] VIII, 84).

From this viewpoint health is nothing but the application of science and technique. It is attainable provided one has invested in the means to do so. As a result the health that society makes available will be regarded as a right which each individual is entitled to claim. This form of depersonalized health, provided obligatorily by society for each of its members, is something they receive from outside with no cost in terms of personal effort. When health and disease are seen only from the viewpoint of scientific medicine and its remedies, we leave far behind the principle which was so dear to Paul Tournier – that health must also be associated with a personal decision, linked often to a fundamental reorientation of one's way of life.

THE OVERWHELMING THIRD

Fascinating and attractive as it can be, this 'third party' can also have aspects which are repulsive, forbidding and overwhelming, particularly in the matter of economic and administrative problems. Without entering into details known to one and all, I must mention today's obsession with finance, the anxiety caused by the omnipresent threat of legal proceedings, and the paralysing effect of a profusion of laws, regulations and directives of every kind.

I believe that we have never previously been so aware of the frightening power of depersonalization of all human organization and of the particular fragility of those who consult us. These very often enter the system of care to say 'enough is enough' in relation to a society in which they feel crushed and suffocated. The system of health care ought to offer them a friendly haven where they can find their feet again and recover their strength. What they look for is not a slavish embodiment of society at large, but rather some detachment from it: they need mediators or even advocates.

Here too the doctor (like all other carers) is in a very ambivalent position. He is a member of the society and by participating in its caring function he is authorized to offer to the sick the support they need. As a member of society the care-giver participates naturally in this positive function, but at the same time he doesn't escape the dangers of technical activism and burdensome bureaucracy. At one and the same time he is society's representative in charge of the patient *and* his advocate in time of need. His open-hearted encounter with a fellow being in distress inevitably leads him not to snap the social bonds that bind him but at least to distance himself from them in a critical spirit. Seeing suddenly before him this person in distress, he will feel compassion to the very core of his being, like the Good Samaritan in the Gospel parable (Luke 10). Alerted by this to the alienation that the 'third party' (society at large) can bring with it, he will seek to stand up against it, not by eliminating the claims of society and seeking refuge in some cosy individual relationship, but by moderating society's promises and requirements. Thus the doctor becomes the patient's champion in his encounter with society. He understands and even shares his revulsion in the face of the supposed or real injustice represented by the disease and its consequences. As for the role of 'sick person' imposed by society (or occasionally self-imposed), the doctor helps him shoulder it and find ways to live with it.

My argument can be summed up as follows: one of the recurring problems in the practice of medicine, and particularly general medicine, is the need to reconcile the strong and inclusive involvement required by the patient with the need to remember always the claims of society at large.

The anecdote at the beginning of this chapter might tempt us to think that the answer lies in choosing one side *against* the other, the patient *against* society at large: we put our feet up and meet for a friendly fireside chat, keeping the fire well stoked up with all those despised papers and administrative documents.

That, however, is a childish attitude – the attempt to deny the existence of something that frightens and distresses us. The same response can be found on the other flank too – people taking refuge in the depersonalized world of administrative necessity or technical complexity through fear of entering into a real personal relationship. The aim of the general practitioner – as heir to the double tradition of personalized care and service to the community – must be to fuse the demands of patient and of the world at large, to argue that they are compatible and that there is no need for one to give way to or be absorbed by the other. What is needed is a constructive interaction between these two aspects of reality, not an artificial war between them. It is in this spirit that the philosopher Paul Ricoeur insists that ethics concerns our relations with ourselves and with others, but in his view this 'search for the good life with and for others' is dependent on 'just institutions' (Ricoeur 1995). It is this notion of justice which I would like now to explore further, aiming to show how it can serve as a link between the two aspects that we want to render compatible – the individual and the collective.

Some notions of justice as a necessity for communal living

There is no need here for a long discussion on justice – just a brief mention of two different ways of viewing it. Stated simplistically, they are two projects for the organization of society, one aiming to maximize the common good of society at large, the other to allow each individual member of society to maximize what is 'good' for himself. There are many other conceptions of justice, but for our purposes it is this tension between the common and the individual good which seems to me particularly relevant.

JUSTICE AS PURSUIT OF THE COMMON GOOD

A classic notion of justice deriving from the ancient philosophers associates it with the recognition and preservation of order in the world and in human society. On this view justice can be said to have at root a collective dimension. This was for example the point of Aristotle's insistence on the fact that, if all virtues have their end in the good of the individual who practises them, the virtue of justice is different in that its end is directed towards the good of the political community. By aiming at a good outside the individual it takes him out of himself and directs him towards other members of the community: 'And it is complete virtue in its fullest sense, because it is the actual exercise of complete virtue. It is complete because he who possesses it can exercise his virtue not only in himself but towards his neighbour also' (Aristotle, *Nicomachean Ethics*, V, 1029b, 30).

We find then in these ancient thinkers the idea of a political community that is more than the simple juxtaposition of isolated individuals each pursuing his own interest. There are in the community itself values that amount to more than the simple sum of those of its constituent members. This means that the search for the common good is something more than the establishment of just relationships between all the possible combinations of pairs of individuals. There is a good that depends on the common functioning of the total community. This being so, the search for justice will have to take into account the character of inter-individual transactions – a necessary component, but of itself insufficient unless complemented by a sense of membership of some larger community for which the individual feels some responsibility. An example from the field of health concerns the prolonged care of distressed and dependent individuals who are at the same time members of the larger community: we should think not simply of the benefit to them as individuals but of the transformation of the whole community, committed thereby to being more open, more tolerant and less elitist.

JUSTICE AS PURSUIT OF WHAT IS GOOD FOR THE INDIVIDUAL

Another conception of justice derives from the idea that society is there only to allow each of its members to enjoy as fully as possible the benefits available to him – above all his freedom. To quote the Roman maxim, justice consists of 'giving to each his due'. The just society must on the one hand distribute available goods equitably, and on the other hand supply the structural framework which will allow each individual the maximum exercise of his freedom. The measure of the common good according to this scheme of things is the scope available to each individual to maximize his benefits and his freedom of action. This is the dominant conception of justice in today's world with its fusion of Western modernity and liberal ideology. Essentially it amounts to a *distributive justice* which specializes in the allocation of resources and makes much of the supporting rationale. Instead of building a social order it limits its aims to the distribution of goods. It focuses on conflicts of interest, which it tries to prevent and resolve by means of procedural frameworks established by consensus.

The notion of a common good implies that the members of a society will have some role in constructing the social order. Thus, insofar as a just society is concerned for the welfare of its sick members and helps them through application of its caring function, it will be generally assumed in return that the good functioning of the community and its progress towards the common good imposes on each individual the *duty of being in good health*. In terms of the definition of good health proposed by the theologian Karl Barth, this involves doing everything possible to retain one's 'capacity to remain human'. By contrast the liberal position stresses much more the notion of *health as a right*: in a just society everyone is entitled to demand it as a right, thereby to maintain maximum personal autonomy and the chance to pursue self-chosen goals.

Theology: a tradition with something to say about communities

Theology has many different ways of enriching the notion of justice, but I want to stress particularly the biblical and theological tradition that makes it an attribute of God. Such a vision of divine justice is bound to give added richness to the justice we seek in a human community. Social organization is not just a matter of procedural management of inter-human relations after applying reason to make the best possible choice. Mention of God's justice implies leaving behind the procedural arrangements whereby each individual receives what is due to him. For unless the God we believe in is fussy and litigious – some super civil servant who gives nothing away without proof of entitlement – we must assume that the justice we attribute to him is compatible with his other attributes (love, tenderness, compassion and the like): something therefore towards which we should strive but with no chance of ever fully achieving it in this world.

There is a permanent unresolved tension here which reminds us that even the most exalting experiences of the life we live is nothing but an imperfect image of the ideal that is our calling. The justice of God's Kingdom as thus conceived, beyond our reach but constantly before us as an ideal, represents a constant challenge to justice conceived on the human level. For this is seen as something attainable on condition that proper institutional management allows individuals actually to achieve the targets they select for their own good.

By contrast the justice that is enriched by divine justice has something to say about a social order but not one where the interactions of separate individuals are regulated by a set of formal rules: it is an order based on perfect fulfilment, on fully harmonious inter-human relations. In the theological tradition this is the brotherhood of man: the notion that all members of the community are 'near and dear' to me personally and that it is for me to register that fact along the lines of the prophet's warning to: '... not hide yourself from your own flesh!' (Isa 58:7).

Brotherhood as membership of the same family is a notion found repeatedly in the Scriptures and the theological tradition. The vision is certainly utopian, but it is rich and fertile in its implications for social relations.

My personal view is that this notion of shared brotherhood takes us beyond the rigid polarity between patient and society at large that we spoke of earlier. Theological utopia suggests that behind theoretical talk of the just distribution of resources, of administrative constraints and budgetary management, there may be something other than a crushing impersonal social machine that puts us on the defensive. Far from distracting us from the priority of concern for our patient-as-brother, the notion of the third-party-as-brother offers a different vision of brotherhood: they are complementary rather than conflicting images insofar as talk of 'family' must imply the sum-total of its members.

In this type of relationship justice must identify each individual's rights but in the context of a concern for all. This goes beyond the liberal concept of justice, whose sole aim is to reduce as far as possible the constraints that the presence or the activities of others might impose upon an individual's liberty.

Psychiatrists tell us that a systematic approach makes it impossible to look after an individual patient without a wider care for the whole family system. Similarly, bearing in mind the notion of a family community within the political body, we could say that one can't look after an individual patient without a concern for the community at large.

Certainly this is a utopian view of things, but utopia (or in theological terms, hope) is what spurs human progress. There is utopia after all in taking a patient for a three-day stay in the mountains: what would happen to general medicine if we made that a general practice? Yet this gesture of Tournier's lives with us as an ideal, and makes us seek to cultivate in relation to each patient the same relational intensity that we perceive in that idealized model. In the same way the notion of justice-as-brotherhood stands before us as both desire and demand – the aim in both cases being to go beyond mere formal procedures to re-impose relational priorities on society at large.

People like Tournier have pushed us – and continue to push us – into prioritizing personal relations in our encounters with individual patients: similarly we are spurred by the theology of justice to extend this relational emphasis to the wider society – to think always of people in their communal context.

General practice: a return to this subject

Let us now try returning to the realities of general practice as we know it: how might the day-to-day business of our surgeries be affected by the vision of things outlined above?

CARE AS A COLLECTIVE PROCESS

It is first of all in the care-givers themselves that one should see a living embodiment of this openness towards the community. Too often we cling to the idea that the doctor presides alone over the caring process. The other professionals or volunteers involved would seem to be there only to facilitate his task and release him from its more tedious aspects so that he can concentrate on his mission of patient care. Breaking down the barrier between the doctor–patient duo and the rest of the world implies that the doctor should recognize his place within a veritable community of carers who bear *as a body* the responsibility for caring despite differences in their training and technical competence. We should always remember that such differences in technical competence are the sole justification for a hierarchical organization of care when maximum effectiveness is the aim. Caring, compassion and companionship to a patient along his road of suffering, these are roles to be taken up by anyone regardless of diplomas, the need often arising in the most unexpected sectors of the caring team. The fact that everyone has a recognized share in the burden of caring breaks down the academic hierarchies and establishes a veritable caring community. A further step is to argue that the caring capacity, being independent of traditional professional training (while benefitting, as it can and should, from systems of apprenticeship), is to be found in society at large. Recognizing this fact implies that looking after another in his need is a communal task with a role for each and everyone, not something limited to the professional community of carers.

AN END TO THE PREOCCUPATION WITH ECONOMICS

If justice is something more than rendering each person his due, its true concern being that we should find a way of living harmoniously with others, then it is of the greatest importance that we should stop drawing a contrast between personal and human face-to-face encounters on the one hand and on the other the economics of relations with society at large. It is true that most of the time, when we think of justice, the things that come to mind are allocation of resources, access to health care for all social categories or the productivity of the provider of health care. We are obsessed these days with the need to master health costs: it is a problem we cannot afford to neglect, but it certainly doesn't deserve our undivided attention. Claiming that the values that count are not uniquely in the economic sphere is not to say that economics disappears from the scene or loses its importance, but simply that it is only one of many aspects of the social context, and not necessarily the most important.

INTERACTION BETWEEN DOCTOR AND COMMUNITY

A doctor who is fully aware of the communal dimension does not 'endure' it like a necessary evil but experiences a constant interaction with it. In particular the fact that he is armed with insight into human relations at their most basic will mean he is called upon to address his fellow men. Such statements may be called for in an intimate context, involving for example relatives in the management of an illness, or in relation to a wider public through speeches, press articles or political debate, where the doctor can draw on his repertoire of unforgettable moments of interaction with patients. To quote an apt remark of Levinas, 'what happens between the two of us is everybody's business'. This does not of course mean a breach of confidentiality, but simply a recognition that the community cannot be left totally unaware of such significant moments in the life of its citizens: they are not only part of the patient's history, but also an enriching element in the history of the community at large. Transmission of this enriching message may often lie with the carer. One thinks here of the incredible number of clinical stories that fill Tournier's books. It is his way of saying that these stories do not belong uniquely to him and to the patient: they are there as a source of enrichment to the world at large.

Think of a doctor who is accompanying a patient through to their death of some chronic disease. His primary concern is naturally the way the patient meets his death and lives his last moments, but of additional importance is the way in which the surrounding family conceive and experience the death, possibly thereby enriching their own conception of death itself. By not refusing to talk about the subject the doctor enables the community in general to be the richer for knowing how a particular individual trod the path through illness to death. The truth is that a society that finds space in its story for disease, disability, dementia or death – ensuring for example that its sick members retain an active role – has a greater social wealth than one which excludes such persons and gives priority to those who suffer no disability.

Conclusion

Walking a few steps with Paul Tournier, as this book would have us do, makes us vividly aware of the fundamental importance of relationships in our caring procedures. His focus on the meeting between the doctor and the patient as the key point in the caring relationship is a precious antidote to those pressures that would distract us from such personal involvement. On the other hand this emphasis is not the whole story and might even lead to an over-concentration on a cosy and exclusive 'solitude for two'. With this in mind I wanted to put in a plea that we should *go beyond a relation-centred perspective and favour a community-centred view.*

This will only, however, deliver the desired benefits on two conditions. First, we must conceive the community itself as a network of rich personal relationships. Second, despite all the doubts and contrary evidence that our real-life experience of humanity might suggest to us, we must strive unfailingly towards that reality which in theology is known as the Kingdom of God. This reality implies deep human face-to-face relationships, which leave nobody excluded: a reality that is mysteriously absent and yet present at the same time; and a reality for a world to come (utopia) yet already present in the here and now. This reality opens us to the complexity of human relations, and asks of us a great modesty when trying to define what is or should be a 'good' doctor–patient relationship. But this should never discourage us from continuously trying to refine our way of being a human presence in front of a suffering person.

References

Arendt, H. (1998 [1958]) *The Human Condition*. Cambridge, MA: University of Chicago Press.

Aristotle (2000 [384–322 BCE]) *Nicomachean Ethics*. Ed/Transl. R. Crisp. Cambridge, Cambridge University Press.

Balint, M. (1957) *The Doctor, his Patient and the Illness*. London: Pitman Medical Publishing.

Buber, M. (1987) *I and Thou*. Edinburgh: T. & T. Clark.

Juvenal (1999 [exact date unknown]) *The Satires*. Transl. N. Nudd. Oxford: Oxford University Press.

Levinas, E. (1969) *Totality and Infinity: An Essay on Exteriority*. Pittsburgh PA: Duquesne University Press.

Ricoeur, P. (1995) *Oneself as Another*. Chicago: University of Chicago Press, Chapter 7.

Tournier, P. (1940) *Médicine de la Personne*. Neuchâtel, Switzerland: Delachaux et Niestlé.

CHAPTER 12

SPIRITUALITY AND CARE: A PUBLIC HEALTH PERSPECTIVE

Tom Fryers

> Although we choose in freedom, we are not independent; for we exercise our freedom in the midst of values and powers we have not chosen but to which we are bound. (Niebuhr 1952, p.247)

Introduction

The 'Medicine of the Person' group has usually been concerned with the individual doctor–patient relationship, but, coming from public health, my perspective is wider than the clinical situation alone. For me, therefore, 'care' includes all those situations common in complex developed societies where professionals, volunteers or family members are caring for others who are sick, frail, disabled, or dying. There is, indeed, a duty of care in all human relations.

I am assuming 'spirituality' to be concerned with components of human life and experience that are not material, nor tangible, but that are unarguably real in every person's life, and give human value and deep satisfaction to that life. For me, these components are largely encompassed by love, joy, peace and faith. Though not essentially intellectual, they will be enhanced by clear and honest thought; though not primarily emotional, they are unlikely to be experienced without feeling. Anything material or social which threatens them prejudices the wholeness, or health, of the person. Anything which fosters them is promoting spiritual healing. They can be experienced in spite of physical or mental suffering, (pain, sickness or disability) but they may enhance the body's healing processes, which diminish physical and mental suffering (Metcalf 1997). Thus body, mind and spirit are inextricably linked in the whole person.

In Christian tradition, love, joy, peace and faith are 'gifts of the Spirit', and are the properties of persons that reveal God within us and within others, and that proclaim the nature of the person beyond the body and the mind, though not apart from the body and the mind. Wakefield writes in his *Dictionary of Spirituality*:

> Christian spirituality is not simply for 'the interior life' or the inward person, but as much for the body as the soul, and is directed to the implementation of both the commandments of Christ: to love God and our neighbour. (Wakefield 1983, p.361)

However, these properties should be conceived as 'spiritual' rather than necessarily 'religious'. Though we might disagree about the means of achieving them, they are equally valid for non-Christians, including people who subscribe to no recognized belief system. And for Christians I am willing to say that they are far more important and fundamental than any particular verbal expression of belief.

Beyond the self

Although they are the properties of persons, they do not represent merely individualistic values. Although it is possible to conceive joy, peace and faith in purely individual terms, or in terms of a purely individual relationship with God, this renders them supremely self-centred, a risk not always avoided by Christian evangelists and apologists. However, love can never be self-centred, which is, presumably, why St Paul says that it is the greatest gift, the greatest quality, both the essence and the fullness of the Spirit-filled life (1 Cor. 13). When joy, peace and faith are informed by love, they too are concerned not only with self but with others.

It should be noted that Jesus endorsed the injunction to 'love your neighbour *as yourself*' (Luke 10:25–28). Loving yourself is not the same as being self-centred. We must feel good about ourselves, and therefore attend to our own deepest needs, if we are to offer ourselves to others to serve their deepest needs. The implication of this is that, in so much as we experience love, joy, peace and faith in our inner lives, they necessarily inform our attitudes, our thinking and our behaviour equally to ourselves and others, in a spiritual unity which is itself an expression of true personal wholeness.

Dominian (1999) writes:

At the heart of love is the process by which we possess ourselves. We cannot be loving – that is, be available to others or to
ourselves – if we do not own ourselves – that is, feel that we are
the possessors of our beings and that we can dispose of ourselves
as we consider fit... What we offer depends on what we feel about
ourselves. If we feel good and lovable, then what we have to offer
will be transmitted in a loving way. (p.130)

Quoist (1965) wrote:

Be yourself. Others need you just as the Lord has willed you to be.
You have no right to put on a false face, to pretend you're what
you're not, unless you want to rob others. Say to yourself: I am going to bring something new into this person's life, because he has
never met anyone like me, nor will he ever meet anyone like me;
for, in the mind of God, I am unique and irreplaceable. (p.51)

Spirituality, therefore, the 'inner life', is a function of individuals, but is
not a merely individualistic phenomenon or experience. If it is an expression of wholeness, it must inevitably overflow to others through all our
relationships, which are the essence and purpose of human existence.

The individual, others and community

Although in the twentieth century we have seen political and quasi-reli-
gious philosophies and systems that, in extreme form, deny individual
personhood and the validity of 'inner life' values, Western European cultures in general have tended, for a long time, to emphasize individual autonomy, reinforced in recent decades by aggressive capitalism and the
political right. In the UK, what became known as 'Thatcherism' emphasized individual autonomous choice, responsibility for your own fate,
economic independence, and societal relationships as competitive or
contractual. Thatcher said 'There is no such thing as society' (Wheen
2004, p.25).

However, the reality of our social existence cannot so readily be denied. Rampant individualism is even more characteristic of dominant
American (US) culture and is the subject of an interesting recent study by
a psychiatrist and a medical ethicist (Gaylin and Jennings 1996) who
quote Reinhold Niebuhr (1944):

Man requires freedom in his social organization because he is "essentially" free, which is to say that he has the capacity for indeterminate transcendence over the processes and limitations of nature… But he also requires community because he is by nature social. He cannot fulfil his life within himself but only in responsible and mutual relations with his fellows.' (p.vi)

The study concludes (*inter alia*), 'Bounded autonomy is a precious human and historical achievement; blanket autonomy is an unsustainable pipe-dream' (Gaylin and Jennings 1996, p.vi).

Even within the Christian Church the same individualism has been evident. Protestant Christian traditions, especially conservative evangelical traditions, also emphasize individual autonomy and focus upon 'my soul to be saved'; 'my personal relationship with God'. Some models of 'Church' may be limited to independent local congregations conceived as groups of saved individuals, and the idea of the Kingdom of God as merely the company of believers.

In societies where such ideas are prevalent, it is very common for people to consider religion, faith and spiritual issues as entirely private matters, not to be discussed with anyone. All views are personal, idiosyncratic and equally justified or valuable. Sex and money are discussed openly and incessantly, but spiritual issues are virtually taboo. If this effectively shuts spiritual issues out of the lives of many people, for them it is as Kierkegaard observed 150 years ago: 'it had become next to impossible to communicate spiritual things directly; people had forgotten what it meant to exist as a human being; they had lost the sense of being spiritual creatures' (Roberts 1957, p.123; Kierkegaard 1941).

In a cultural context such as this, it is not easy for professionals in any care situation to enter into 'inner life' issues unless they know their client well, they themselves have confronted issues of spirituality, healing and wholeness in their own lives, and they have, for themselves, conquered the taboo on discussing them.

However, most of us live in societies that are not extreme. Although very individualistic and competitive in general culture, there is also a widespread commitment to provide for those in need within the community, especially in education, health and social support. The degree to which the welfare state and charitable agencies are developed varies between different countries, but most Western European countries experience the dilemmas involved. The economics of communal support ('welfare') for children, the sick, disabled people, the unemployed and the elderly pose huge challenges for every developed society and it is inappropriate to attempt to deal with such issues here.

Nevertheless, it seems to me that to ensure that poverty, sickness and disability in our societies are dealt with in an organized, disciplined, just, and reliable way as communal action expresses love – 'inner life' values of compassion, brotherliness, sensitivity and humility – in a highly practical way which is impossible if left entirely to individual action. Moreover it can be done without blaming people who are victims of individual misfortune or societal change, or challenging their self respect or the respect of others. The Kingdom of God, which Jesus said 'has come upon us' (Mark 1:15; Luke 11:20), though not to be equated with any earthly organization or social system, surely encompasses all actions of love, compassion, healing and care, evidence of the Holy Spirit's current and eternal involvement with all human history, all cultures, all people: 'The manifest and effective assertion of the divine sovereignty against all the evil of the world' (Dodd 1935, p.59). It is possible for social organizations providing care to the sick, the disabled and the dying to mediate this on a broad scale even where many individuals involved are not themselves Christians.

Givers and receivers of care

I wish to focus on a dilemma which is more personally concerned with 'inner life' values of people who are in need of, and in receipt of 'care'. Care may be a simple consultation with a doctor, but in our complex modern health and social service systems it often involves many professionals. Care also often involves non-professional carers within families and communities, who may indeed carry most of the burden of care. The issue concerns 'dependence', which can be viewed from two different perspectives.

First, 'welfare' systems, whether mediated by the state, by a charitable agency or by an individual professional, are often perceived as fostering dependence upon 'authority' or the agents of 'authority'. These agents might include doctors, especially for people with long-term or frequent illness who are well known to their doctors, but often also for people who have serious personal and interpersonal problems, or who are lonely, unemployed, in poverty or in other stressful circumstances, many of whom seek a doctor's attention and many of whom are depressed or anxious.

Depression and anxiety are extremely common. Statistics from the UK (Mann 1992) suggest that demonstrable psychosocial difficulties are present in one third of all people who attend for a General Practice medical consultation. The annual prevalence of depression and anxiety in adults is 15–25 per cent, depending on clinical criteria; 60–70 per cent of adults will at some time experience depression or anxiety sufficiently severe to interfere with daily activities. The UK National Household Psychiatric Surveys of 1993 (and 2000), providing some of the most reliable measures of any research (Meltzer *et al.* 1995; Singleton *et al.* 2001), found 12.6 per cent (14.4%) of men and 19.9 per cent (20.2%) of women aged 16–64 years to have had a recognizable neurotic disorder within one week of the interview, using standard assessments (CIS-R). When we recognize that depression and anxiety are often associated with significant life events and restricting and stigmatizing social circumstances, it is not surprising that doctors and health care systems have commonly to deal with social and economic issues including all aspects of 'dependence'.

Second, and in the same cultural context, it is common to hear complaints from patients about being dependent, not only economically, but in terms of mobility, personal care, access to services, and so on. This perception is common among disabled people with significant disadvantages in society, but who have engendered powerful self-help organizations, the disabled rights movements and a substantial industry of disability aids to confront dependence. It is prominent among elderly people whose capacity to act independently is gradually deteriorating and who feel powerless to combat dependence. It is a source of low self-esteem and depression in unemployed people and single mothers and their children.

From both perspectives, avoiding unnecessary dependence has, for many years, been a major object of health care and of preventive medicine (Susser and Watson 1971) and 'dependence' has become a very negative word and concept. In our cultures the ideal life is portrayed as one of total independence; the whole person is perceived as wholly autonomous. Anyone who cannot fulfil this expectation may be stigmatized and devalued. However, there is one exception, that is, in traditional health care, (which is, of course, largely 'sickness care'), where the 'sick role' is accepted without loss of respect from self or others (Parsons 1951). Because this is the one significant general exception, there is inevitably a tendency to call anything 'sickness' if there is a perceived need to permit dependence without loss of self-esteem.

As a consequence, we may create expectations of 'treatment' and hopes of 'cure' within a medical model, which may inhibit both patient and doctor from facing up to the realities of the patient's situation, whether the primary issues are economic, social or spiritual. This 'medicalization' of personal problems has long been recognized. It poses particular difficulties in psychiatry where it remains problematic (for example) to discriminate serious disorders to which it is legitimate to apply an illness model, from normal reactions to abnormal situations or experiences, and extreme variations of human personality (Goldberg and Huxley 1992). Where psychoanalytical approaches to therapy were appropriate, it could have a positive image, though dependence upon the therapist was a well recognized phenomenon. But sociological analysis of the vast majority of medical contexts gave 'medicalization' a largely negative image. Because depression and anxiety are so common, it is easy to confuse, conceal or deny spiritual problems such as disordered relationships, low self-esteem, guilt and fear by diagnosing a depressive illness and treating it with medication.

It is common to blame the medical profession for this situation, but the responsibility is shared throughout society. There is collusion between doctors, patients, health systems and society at large; a collective dishonesty in the cause of legitimizing dependency. It has been argued that we need other models comparable to the sick role, such as a 'disabled role' or a 'frail elderly role'. But, unlike the sick role, these roles would generally be permanent, there would be little expectation of recovery, and most people in the groups concerned do not wish to be dependent! In any case, deeply entrenched societal perceptions are not easily changed; the sick role was an observation, not a creation of the sociologists!

Interdependence and reciprocity

From a spiritual perspective the problem might be analysed and its solution approached in a different way. It seems to me as a doctor and a Christian that we need to conceive human life in terms not of autonomy or dependence, but in terms of interdependence. Each individual needs both separate identity and close relationships, neither controlled by other people, or lost in another's personality, nor set against everyone else in competition, but living in rich interdependence with others, and acknowledging the contribution, genetic, cultural and environmental, of human society to his or her assumptions, beliefs, expectations and experiences.

The ideal is, perhaps, a loving acceptance of each other as we are, and a joyful tension between individual creative thought and action, cultural norms and physical limitations. This might indeed generate peace of mind and heart for the present, and faith in the future that transcends pain, suffering, loss, sickness and death. The life of Jesus might be interpreted in these terms.

Even our relationship with God can be viewed somewhat in contrast to traditional theological formulations that emphasize our total dependence upon Him as one of interdependence: He first creates us free with free will, then recreates us free through forgiveness and the Spirit's indwelling, to relate to Him by choice, as 'friends not servants' (John 15:14/15) and to get on with His work on earth, for which He is largely dependent upon us.

In the practice of care we can promote such interdependence, whether we work in general medical practice, psychiatry, psychology, social work, or other caring professions, or we are involved in caring for others as a neighbour or within our own family. If we are to make a contribution, we will need to have dealt with these spiritual issues for ourselves, and will need to be clear-headed in our objectives for others. Freeling, a Professor of General Practice, wrote in a professional context: 'The GP needs not only social and interpersonal skills, but, most important, self-knowledge' (1992, p.64). One of the most encouraging developments during a year spent in Bosnia with the World Health Organization (WHO) after the fighting had been brought to an end was the commitment of General Medical Practitioners in Sarajevo to a Balint group programme which emphasized self-knowledge, reconciliation and healing for themselves as well as their patients.

I will deal with aspects of the relationship between carer and cared-for under six headings:

1. caring is sharing

2. caring acknowledges the whole person

3. receiving is also to be blessed

4. a ministry of reconciliation

5. process and outcomes

6. whole persons live in communities.

CARING IS SHARING

There is a long tradition in Western medicine of the authoritarian doctor, at worst unfeelingly dictatorial, at best paternalistic. 'The doctor must be on his guard: he is used to giving orders' (Tournier 1957, p.201). The doctor is considered to have command of all relevant information, generally has a superior social status, and can exploit the accepted sick role to exercise unquestioned authority. This used to be common, but at least in the UK, it is now relatively rare. In *Creative Suffering*, Tournier (1982, p.47) described the dilemma of doctors facing dying patients: 'Great progress has been made since I was a student. Then we simply had to take refuge in lies.' I can say the same thing. Since I was a student in the 1950s, doctors have become far more honest and open, far more willing to reveal the diagnosis and prognosis to patients and to discuss options for intervention and action, though few, I think, venture into spiritual issues.

Through developments in psychology, psychotherapy, social case work and counselling, there is also a non-directive tradition in which the patient or client makes his or her own choices for treatment or other action. The professional role is only to inform, guide and facilitate. This is widely discussed in the media and promoted by 'patient rights' groups as a model for all medical care.

The first tradition creates total dependence, only justified, perhaps, for surgeons while patients are under the anaesthetic! The second leaves the whole burden of decision-making on the person in need, who, in technical matters at least, can rarely be truly *fully* informed and whose sickness, suffering or impairment may seriously affect their capacity to make decisions. Doctors and other care professionals need to find a balance through an open, therapeutic relationship and with wise judgement.

Establishing and maintaining a secure individual identity is important. If a child does not do this, aspects of immaturity affect his capacity to fulfil his potential as an adult. But I believe that it has been damaging to conceive this as growing into total autonomy, total independence of parents. The ideal is to grow into adult relationships of mutual interdependence between parents and their offspring. Perhaps this is happening more frequently now, as the formal authority of parents has generally diminished; it is not uncommon for adult children to share ongoing interests and activities with their parents, but I'm not sure that is yet the norm. The process of allowing children progressive autonomy while gradually developing relationships of equality is far from easy.

Of course, it is not only parent–child relationships that can go wrong. It is also possible for a person to be totally dominated by a husband or wife, and for their own personality to be lost in the relationship. This is recognizably not a healthy adult relationship. Tournier said 'The result is lamentable – it is no longer a marriage!'(1957, p.225). And sometimes the parent–child relationship is reversed in later years with a son or daughter dominating an unequal and unhealthy relationship with an aging parent. In the twenty-first century, with our aging populations, it is common to see very old people, not in extreme circumstances, treated as totally dependent by professional or family carers, so that they even see themselves as totally dependent.

I think it wrong (in spite of Shakespeare in *As You Like It!*) to call very old age 'second childhood'; it is neither similar nor comparable except in very stigmatizing features. It is often a period of limited learning, growth and development, which are the essence of childhood, and is characterized by long and deep experience impossible in childhood. Older people need to continue to contribute to others from their store of knowledge, skills and experience. In the sharing of the care relationship, it is necessary to recognize and facilitate expression of that experience which, even in technology-dominated societies, can offer interest, education and wisdom to others. Of course there are extreme situations which preclude this, particularly with dementia, but this does not apply to the vast majority.

The professional in the care situation usually has the initiative, having wider professional knowledge and experience than the patient or client, and should have a clear and dispassionate mind to apply to the situation. It is, therefore, primarily the professional's responsibility to get the balance right between facilitating independent decisions and actions and being prescriptive and directive on the patient's behalf. This calls for true wisdom in professional relationships, whether in a traditional consultation between patient and doctor concerning sickness, or in caring for an elderly person in a domestic setting. And it is best done where there is a real sharing of yourself as well as your knowledge and time and, where appropriate, as much of your inner self as the patient can receive (Tournier 1982).

CARING ACKNOWLEDGES THE WHOLE PERSON

We know that many people consulting a doctor have broader and deeper needs than the overt reason for their consultation would suggest. Of particular importance are the spiritual needs concerning self-esteem, relationships with others and relationship with God. Good doctors with a perception of whole person care will often recognize this and will want to offer help at a deeper level. However, few, even in psychiatry, will be able to do this very often in normal practice. We all work with practical constraints of time, economics, technologies and organizations, constraints shared by all other care professionals.

This situation requires not only spiritual qualities but clear thinking and good management:

1. Many people in consultation have relatively simple needs, simply met. The most efficient and effective doctor is able to discriminate these from those for whom he needs more time.

2. He must be able to supply those simple needs with kindness and care, revealing his own spirituality, his own perception that the person is far more than a diseased body or a disordered organ, even where spiritual issues are not the current concern of this patient.

3. If the doctor wishes to offer help in spiritual matters, he must ensure that he has appropriate psychological and spiritual training. Even in 1934, Weatherhead, a pioneer in relating psychology and religion, said, 'The patient must be understood. If we haven't – and we haven't – Christ's insight, we must learn how to look deeply into the mind by scientific methods and then apply the required truth (for example, forgiveness)' (p.30). With the growth of knowledge and technology, the potential and therefore the need for training is far greater now.

4. The doctor needs to make sure that his practice is organized to permit him to give time when he judges it appropriate. For most people in current practice this means agreeing all sorts of practical matters with colleagues and explaining what your approach is. Expressing your spiritual values in relationships with your colleagues may be more difficult than in relationships with your patients!

5. The doctor must recognize that he may not be the right person to explore spiritual issues with a particular patient and must be willing to refer. And he may need to get involved in wider health service organizational matters to ensure that there will be appropriate people to whom he can refer. In the UK in recent years, the greatest need expressed by general practitioners has been for counsellors to work in the practice as a member of the primary care team, resulting in a

rapid expansion in their numbers. Although the development has been unplanned and varied, early evaluation suggests that many patients are aware that physical illness is not the main issue 'and they are not at all surprised to be offered counselling rather than other forms of medical treatment' (Manzi 1992, p.87). This is encouraging.

RECEIVING IS ALSO TO BE BLESSED

Those who complain about being dependent, whether in sickness, disability or very old age, may have much to give that needs to be discovered, but they, like the rest of us, need also to learn how to receive gratefully and gracefully. When Paul reported Jesus as saying, 'It is more blessed to give than to receive' (Acts 20:35), it is obvious what he meant in terms of a Christian life of sacrificial service. Yet in his own life Jesus showed us also how to receive hospitality and other loving ministrations from the hands of others. The woman who poured expensive ointment over him was commended because it was offered in love (Mark 14:3–9; John 12:3–8).

The teaching of Jesus emphasized receiving from God before we can give back our lives in service. You must accept help in getting rid of the plank out of your own eye before you can help remove the speck out of your brother's eye (Matt. 7:3–5). Peter had to accept Jesus washing his feet or he could not be in fellowship with him (John 13:6–9). This was against all Peter's instincts of commitment, service and pride. Not for nothing has pride always been considered the chief sin.

It is common in Western societies for people to resent being in a position of receiving without being able to pay back in some immediate and tangible way. Some time ago I worked with a new colleague in a developing country, in which we were given hospitality everywhere, and gifts from many people. She was perpetually distressed because she had not brought gifts for them and was not allowed to pay for hospitality, and tried persistently to refuse every new offering. Our hosts were expressing their love for us and their thanks for what we were trying to do for their communities. In the same way, many people receiving care feel resentful at being dependent and need to be helped to see the receiving of services in a positive way, to accept them in peace and with joy.

Modern Western societies do tend to focus upon a type of commercial relationship in which reciprocity is immediate. You pay for things now, or you give some service in return to the same person and soon. But human communities do not only work like that. When our children were small, my wife had to ferry older ones to and from school while caring for the younger ones at home. A friend whose children were all at school offered to include ours in her school trips; my wife was thankful but expressed the reservation that she would never be in a position to do the same thing for her in return. Our friend replied that that is not how the world works; 'You', she said, 'will do other things for other people at other times.'

This is ultimately the key to reciprocity. We serve where and when others need us; we receive where and when we are in need. The relationship spreads over the whole community and over a whole lifetime. When we are well, when we are young, when we are well off, we give more than we receive; when we are sick, when we are old, when we are poor, we receive more than we give. The balance is held within the whole community; do not worry about your individual account as long as you are at peace. If we could help others to see their lives in this way, there would be less stress, less anxiety, more peace, more joy, and more self-esteem among those whose experience of sickness, suffering and frailty is compounded by their inability to receive graciously and be blessed. We all need to learn to accept gifts of love with joy, and go in peace.

A MINISTRY OF RECONCILIATION

If pride prevents people from accepting gifts, how much more does it prevent people from accepting and offering forgiveness? Not just big things, but all the little everyday things for which we need forgiveness. 'Love can be defined as staying in relationship, and forgiveness is an essential component of staying in relationship' (Dominion 1999, p.160).

The inner life is disturbed whenever we are in conflict with others. People seeking help for depression and anxiety, for psychosomatic disorders, for intangible general complaints, may have disturbed relationships in the background of their sickness. But it is wider than this, for disturbed relationships can affect people's capacity to work and to live at peace with their neighbours. And for people who are approaching death, whether in old age or not, reconciliation to those with whom they have passed their lives is a high priority if they are to have peace. Jewell (1999) has written:

> Older people will frequently confess that their deepest desire is to die at peace; with their fellows, with their God, and therefore with themselves. The damage and the hurts we inflict on one another as human beings cry out for resolution even though they may lie buried deep in the psyche. The unfinished business of human relationships from our earlier years becomes the pressing business of our later years. (p.11)

In this we recognize the demands of justice in our relationships, which can only be fulfilled in love. Tillich, in his study *Love, Power, and Justice* (1954), said:

> The relation of justice to love in personal encounters can adequately be described through three functions of creative justice, namely: listening, giving and forgiving. In none of them does love do more than justice demands, but in each of them love recognizes what justice demands. (p.84)

In any care situation in which it is possible to enter into spiritual issues, this matter of reconciliation must be dealt with, and professionals dealing with it will inevitably be brought face to face with their own relationships and their own need for reconciliation. In the complexity of our modern professional and personal lives, it is far from easy to resolve all the inadequate and spoilt relationships within our families, with neighbours and colleagues, with transitory contacts, with people with whom we have lost touch, with some who have died. Any such unresolved conflicts may affect our inner lives.

Resolution theoretically must involve the other person, but it is not always possible, and we may be able to do much of it only through our relationship with God, through his forgiveness and his acceptance. In one of his sermons Tillich (1962) wrote:

> Sometimes…it is as though a voice were saying: 'You are accepted; *you are accepted*, accepted by that which is greater than you, … Simply accept the fact that you are accepted!' If that happens, we experience grace,…everything is transformed. In that moment grace conquers sin, and reconciliation bridges the gulf of estrangement. (p.163)

PROCESS AND OUTCOMES

The Methodist Covenant Service is the one unique contribution of Methodism to Christian liturgy. As part of our covenant with God, it includes the commitment to accept being 'laid aside' for God as well as being 'employed' for God (*Methodist Worship Book* 1999). For many people, being laid aside in sickness, disability or old age, unable to work or to achieve, is a great burden. This is especially so in cultures where work, achievement and success represent the highest values in society. I do not know if the 'Protestant work ethic' is only characteristic of Britain and the USA, but the worship of economic and social success is certainly far wider. There is much good in this, but people need also to be able to accept periods in their lives when they cannot pursue success and cannot work for achievements of the kind most readily recognized by society.

Professionally, we are increasingly being driven towards the practice of 'evidence-based medicine' and health care, and this is right. So much practice has had insufficient evidence for its efficacy and cost-effectiveness, which are ethical imperatives in modern technological medicine wherever possible. But they are not always possible. There are areas of practice where we do not yet know enough scientifically to evaluate our interventions, as in much mental health practice. The ethical imperative there is to conduct high quality research.

But there are also aspects of practice where the approach is inappropriate, especially where spiritual values are concerned. Although there is increasing evidence that effective social support, and expressed compassion through comforting, encouraging, calming and praying, can increase the likelihood and speed of recovery from many illnesses, and may prevent illness after adverse life events, probably through immunological mechanisms (Metcalf 1997), and, of course, we would always like to see demonstrable improvements in patients' lives, our interventions should not always depend upon results as conventionally measured. In personal encounters in which the whole person is fully recognized, love, compassion, giving and forgiving are called for in all cases. The application of love in caring relationships places *process* above *outcomes, means* above *ends.*

This means that *being* is similarly placed above *doing.* For technological medicine the doctor needs to be as well trained and as technically competent as possible. But considering spiritual aspects of the relationship between doctor and patient, being a loving person is more important than anything he or she does. We might recall what Pascal wrote in the 'Pensees': 'People should not be able to say of anyone that he is a mathematician, or a preacher, or an eloquent man, but that he is a *man.*' And: 'What I need is a *man* who can fill all my wants at the same time.' (41, 1961 [1669], p.40)

WHOLE PERSONS LIVE IN COMMUNITIES

Earlier I emphasized the communal aspects of human life, even of the inner life. There are very practical implications in relation to 'care'. Christians working for development agencies in poor communities must accept the primacy of loving care and practical service where overt Christian preaching raises hostility in the community and prejudices the development work itself. I have seen this happen. Mature Christians in such work take a wider and longer perspective. God is interested in the whole person and the whole of his life, and their Christian ministry is to serve very needy people whatever their needs are – economic, environmental, agricultural, medical, educational or spiritual. Love cannot deny the wholeness of persons, and cannot deny the reality of communities.

If we are prompted by our own spiritual values to view with compassion the poverty of so many people in the world, we must recognize that the most effective action involves long-term development and preventive programmes at the community level, so that people can establish, communally, the means of feeding, clothing, educating and healing themselves. Needy individuals are frequently the product of needy communities. And small communities throughout the world are increasingly linked by a mutual interdependence in trade, travel, conflict, environmental change and other ways. We must recognize that interdependence; offering care to people in the poorest countries may include, for example, advocacy to our own governments towards cancelling those countries' burden of international debt.

Even at the individual level, for some people presenting with medical symptoms, but appearing to have deeper spiritual needs, we may have first to deal with practical economic, employment or housing issues. And if this is our spiritual response to an individual's need, then the same spiritual promptings may lead us to get involved in community action, even political action, to address such issues on a larger scale. Goldberg, addressing issues of mental illness, wrote: 'Preventive interventions are mainly sociopolitical… Politicians and educators are the key players… Our job is to remind them of the evidence' (Goldberg 1998, p.13). And Caplan (1964), one of the earliest advocates of preventive psychiatry, took great encouragement from President Kennedy's bold Message to Congress of 1963 because he believed it emphasized 'that henceforward the prevention, treatment, and rehabilitation of the mentally ill and the mentally retarded are to be considered a community responsibility and not a private problem' (p.3).

Since people are 'whole persons' and their whole-personhood is tied in to relationships, cultures and communities, their needs are inevitably broad and complex, and a commitment to care is a challenge offering both excitement and risks. It is certainly true that where communities break down dramatically, many individuals are seriously disturbed and in deep personal need, as we have seen in Bosnia and in Kosovo. The Old

Testament is the story of God's dealings with a community. Ultimately our aims must include not only wholeness for persons, but also wholeness for communities, which must often be a painful and protracted process. There are so many hurt bodies, hurt minds, hurth souls, so many disturbed or destroyed relationships, and we cannot achieve much alone. As Desmond Tutu said in an African prayer called 'Reflections on Wholeness' (1995): 'Our wholeness is intertwined with their hurt. / Wholeness means healing the hurt, working with Christ to heal the hurt, / Seeing and feeling the suffering of others, standing alongside them' (p.110).

Conclusion

I have ranged fairly widely and will not attempt to sum up. To be involved in medical practice and health care is a great privilege. To have the opportunity of facilitating others towards wholeness is a high calling. I will close simply with another word from Desmond Tutu's prayer: 'We yearn to experience wholeness in our innermost being;/Our spirits cry out for the well-being of the whole human family' (p.110).

God, who gives us strength of body, mind and spirit, make us whole.

Acknowledgement

An earlier version of this paper was first given at the 1999 Annual meeting of the Association European Médecine de la Personne, Bischof Bennohaus, Schmochtitz, Bautzen, FRG, July.

References

Caplan, G. (1964) *Principles of Preventive Psychiatry.* London: Tavistock.

Dodd, C.H. (1935) *The Parables of the Kingdom.* London: James Nisbet.

Dominian, J. (1999) *One Like Us: A Psychological Interpretation of Jesus.* London: Dartman, Longman and Todd.

Freeling, P. (1992) 'Implications for General Practice Training and Education.' In R. Jenkins, J. Newton and R. Young (eds) *The Prevention of Depression and Anxiety; The Role of the Primary Care Team.* London: HMSO.

Gaylin, W. and Jennings, B. (1996) *The Perversion of Autonomy.* New York: Free Press.

Goldberg, D. and Huxley, P. (1992) *Common Mental Disorders: a Bio-Social Model.* London: Routledge.

Goldberg, D. (1998) 'Prevention of Mental Illness.' In R. Jenkins and T.B. Ustun (eds) *Preventing Mental Illness: Mental Health Promotion in Primary Care.* Chichester: Wiley.

Jewell, A. (1999) *Introduction, Spirituality and Ageing.* London: Jessica Kingsley.

Kierkegaard, S. (1941) *Concluding Unscientific Postscript.* Princeton: Princeton University Press.

Mann, A. (1992) 'Depression and Anxiety in Primary Care: The Epidemiological Evidence.' In R. Jenkins, J. Newton and R. Young (eds) *The Prevention of Depression and Anxiety: The Role of the Primary Care Team.* London: HMSO.

Manzi, C. (1992) 'Counselling in General Practice; Options for Action: Person-Centred Counselling.' In R. Jenkins, J. Newton and R. Young (eds) *The Prevention of Depression and Anxiety: The Role of the Primary Care Team.* London: HMSO.

Meltzer, H., Gill, B., Pettigrew, M. and Hinds, K. (1995) *The Prevalence of Psychiatric Morbidity Among Adults Living in Private Households.* GB Psychiatric Surveys, Report 1. London: OPCS.

Metcalf, D. (1997) *A Mechanism for Miracles.* Unpublished paper to Methodist Synod, Cumbria District.

Methodist Worship Book (1999) London: Methodist Publishing House.

Niebuhr, R. (1944) *The Children of Light and the Children of Darkness.* New York: Scribner's Sons.

Niebuhr, R. (1952) *Christ and Culture.* London: Faber.

Parsons, T. (1951) *The Social System.* New York: Free Press.

Pascal, B. (1961 [1669]) *The Pensees.* Transl. J.M. Cohen. London: Penguin.

Quoist, M. (1965) *The Christian Response.* Dublin: Gill and Macmillan.

Roberts, D.E. (1957) *Existentialism and Religious Belief.* New York: OUP (Galaxy).

Singleton, N., Bumpstead, R., O'Brien, M., Lee, A. and Meltzer, H. (2001) *Psychiatric Morbidity Among Adults Living in Private Households, 2000.* London: The Stationary Office.

Susser, M.W. and Watson, W. (1971) *Sociology in Medicine,* 2nd edn. London: OUP.

Tillich, P. (1954) *Love, Power and Justice.* New York: OUP (Galaxy).

Tillich, P. (1962) *The Shaking of the Foundations.* London: Penguin.

Tournier, P. (1957) *The Meaning of Persons.* London: SCM Press.

Tournier, P. (1982) *Creative Suffering.* London: SCM Press.

Tutu, D. (1995) *An African Prayer Book.* London: Hodder and Stoughton.

Wakefield, G.S. (1983) 'Spirituality.' In C.S. Wakefield (ed) *A Dictionary of Christian Spirituality.* London: SCM Press.

Weatherhead, L.D. (1934) *Psychology and Life.* London: Hodder and Stoughton.

Wheen, F. (2004) *How Mumbo-Jumbo Conquered the World.* London: Harper Perennial.

CHAPTER 13

THE RE-EMERGENCE OF HOME HEALTH CARE: A HOLISTIC RESPONSE TO AGING AND CONSUMER EMPOWERMENT

Mike Magee

Introduction

The health care system in the USA has quietly evolved on multiple fronts over the past two decades. Health consumers are increasingly educated and empowered. Health now implies overall wellbeing and the opportunity to reach one's full human potential, rather than disease intervention or the health system itself. Physicians have moved away from paternalism and are embracing partnerships with patients and team formation to support both clinical continuums and real-time education. Broadband service is now in the majority of physicians' offices and patients' homes, and the Internet continues to grow as a source of health information. There is a renewed policy focus on safety, evidence, and equity translated into examinations of hospital processes, exploration of the fragmented safety net, and sorting out of class-versus-race contributors to health disparities. An insurance approach that has conspired to restrict patient access to care-givers, and restrict choice of therapies, is being soundly rejected. Most patients now understand the major chronic diseases and their causes, and are beginning to absorb the concepts of lifespan management, with women (as usual) leading the way.

The USA may have accomplished much in the last 20 years, but has yet to successfully convert its system from an emphasis on intervention to prevention, has yet to resolve the large numbers of uninsured citizens, and has yet to fully leverage information systems and technology to strengthen the patient–physician relationship and reinforce multi-generational health. Yet hidden in the current converging mega-trends are predictable tipping points that, in the near future, will quietly transform health care around a home-centric holistic model better able to provide health for the person.

Challenges of aging

However, is good health simply delaying the inevitable, a long and expensive deterioration occurring later in life? Surprisingly, no. Studies of centenarians have shown that their decades of relative good health are followed by a highly compressed period of compromised health at the end of life (Perls 1997).

Donna Shalala, Commissioner of Health and Human Services at the turn of the twentieth century, said:

> We want life not only to be long, but good. This will be one of the central challenges of the twenty-first century: to make dignity and comfort for the elderly as much a part of our national consciousness as education and safety are for our children. (Shalala 1999)

We are in a scientific and social service race against the very real challenges of aging demographics. There is therefore a need for a two-pronged strategy. The first arm is enlightened prevention and health maintenance, intended to help elders maintain vitality and independence for as long as possible, by aggressively addressing those conditions that lead to disability and institutionalization. The second arm, which is complementary to the first, is the creation of new environments that actively manage the changes and disabilities that come with advanced age.

Long-term care is part of the natural fabric of life. It is fundamentally different from acute care in that it integrates health services and supports daily living. The explosive growth of the long-term care industry in the USA simply reflects the numbers, with a projected doubling of the over-65s and tripling of the over-85s in the next 50 years (Administration Association for Homes and Services for the Aging [AAHSA] 1999). During this period, the number requiring long-term care in the USA is projected to grow from under 10 million to 24 million. We should not confuse our future vision of long-term care, however, with old images of restrictive nursing homes.

Activities of daily living

What is it that causes individuals to require this support? The need for long-term care is measured by the limitation in capacity to perform certain basic functions or activities called 'activities of daily living,' or ADLs. ADLs include bathing, dressing, getting in and out of bed, eating, toileting, and moving about. There are other activities, called 'instrumental activities of daily living,' or IADLs, such as getting out, driving, preparing meals, shopping, maintaining a home, using a phone, managing finances and taking medications, which are critical and require help if absent, though not on the level of absent ADLs.

Most of those requiring long-term care prefer to 'age in place,' in their own home and community, in familiar settings. And most do just that. In fact, the use of nursing homes in the USA is declining in all categories of aging, with numbers of nursing home patients over 85 declining by nearly 10 per cent between 1985 and 1995 (Bishop 1999). Instead, what we see is nearly 90 per cent of seniors living in their own homes, independently or with informal care that is almost always provided by family or close friends. This compares with 4.5 per cent who are living at home with professional care and 4.6 per cent residing in nursing homes (van Nostrand, Clark and Romoren 1993).

The race against the aging juggernaut, then, is about science, about independence, and about 'aging in place.' Long-term care is rapidly evolving with a primary focus on dignity, personal autonomy, and support for care-givers.

Trends in long-term care

What are the major trends in long-term care?

1. Less institutionalized care. Nursing homes are being reserved for the most severely impaired.

2. More reliance on home care and community-based alternatives. Day-care options, blended services, 'assisted living,' and care for the care-giver programmes all signal a shift in emphasis that presages a shift in finances.

3. These environments will feature more choices, greater use of supportive new life-assist technologies, a greater emphasis on prevention, and the opportunity for shared learning and community-based strategic planning.

If one were to plan, what might emerge as the best environment for mature living? It would be a place that supports dignity and privacy, one that balances personal autonomy with safety, a place that leverages technology to enhance personal security and safety, one that provides stimulation and social interaction, and assures easy access to affordable services.

There is a great deal of work to be done to get ahead of the aging curve. But we should be optimistic for two reasons. The solution relies on the goodness of individuals, families and communities on the one hand, and on the power of innovation imbedded in our global scientific and medical enterprise on the other.

Informal care-givers: under stress

Home care of dependent, frail seniors falls predominantly on third-generation women aged 45 to 65, attending to parents and/or grandparents as well as to children and grandchildren. Caught in between, they struggle to manage up and down the generation divide. In the USA family and friends provide 80 per cent of long-term care (Havens 1990). The inability to adequately address chronic disease insures organ damage and disability. This cycle has created the 'The Sandwich Generation', squeezed between children and grandchildren on the right, and parents and grandparents on the left. In addition to these care-givers' inability to prevent and treat their own disease, the cost includes reduced ability to contribute to the workforce; a resource/time and financial burden; and increasingly the hidden costs of depression, stress and anxiety.

Colliding mega-trends are increasingly pitting family loyalties against workplace loyalties. As the population has aged, families have become more mobile, separated by distance, and occupied by work demands. Large numbers of women have entered the workplace, and global competitiveness has placed increasing emphasis on worker retention and productivity. Thus, family care-giving from a distance has become a fact of life for millions of Americans.

Care-givers with jobs outside of the home are often required to make significant adjustments to allow for their care-giving responsibilities. These include coming in late or leaving early, missing days of work, rearranging work schedules, and taking unpaid leave. The forces that have created today's long-distance care-giver realities are unlikely to reverse themselves in the near future. Rather, the challenges and work-balance issues are likely to accelerate.

But that's only what you see. Here's what you don't see. The rates of depression in care-givers are significant. Fully 43 per cent of care-givers of Alzheimer patients in one study were clinically depressed (Schultz, Mendelsohn, Haley *et al.* 2003), and only the death of the patient brings lasting relief. Of these care-givers 17 per cent require anti-depressant medicine and 19 per cent require anti-anxiety medications. These rates do not decline if the patient is placed in a nursing home, leaving the family care-giver to struggle with the guilt of abandonment, concerns over institutional care, and bereavement for a loved one who is lost but not gone. It is only after a patient dies, with an average of 3 to 12 months of recovery, that depression levels in family care-givers decline to below the levels of depression that existed when they were active care-givers (Schultz *et al.* 2003).

It is clear that patients prefer to be at home, yet care-givers receive no mental relief by providing home care. What can be done? The solution lies in better systems for home-based support for patients and care-givers. This has the potential to increase quality of care and decrease cost of care. Experts suggest these services focus on five key areas: communication techniques, pain control, vigilance or oversight of wandering behaviour, counselling and positive reinforcement for care-givers, and team-based long-term support (Ory, Hoffman, Yee *et al.* 1999).

What can an employer do? Certainly, sensitizing line managers to the issue is a reasonable starting point. Adjusting policies to allow job sharing and short-time relief, as well as providing information and help in co-ordinating eldercare, are definitely worthwhile investments, compared to the cost of attrition and lost productivity. And, since long-distance care-givers have financial burdens as well as time conflicts, programmes that offer help with these are beneficial. For example, voluntary pooling of frequent flyer miles for employees who need to travel on family emergencies is an idea worth considering (MetLife and National Alliance for Care-giving 2004). These tangible expressions of support face the issue head on while reinforcing shared values and joint commitment.

STRESSED CARE-GIVERS
How are care-givers reacting to the time, workplace, mental and financial constraints of the new reality? They are leading the consumer empowerment movement. Educational empowerment and direct consumer engagement are increasingly the rule. As patients are placed at clinical and financial risk for their decisions, physicians are restructuring to create

both clinical and educational teams with patients and family care-givers themselves as team members.

These dynamics are now reshaping the patient–physician relationship. Studies in the USA and around the world show marked changes in the patient–physician relationship over the past 20 years. Paternalistic relationships are no longer embraced by either doctor or patient. They have been replaced by mutual partnership models and a growing emphasis on clinical and educational team support. Over 90 per cent of doctors now believe the best patient is an educated patient. Patients are increasingly emancipated, empowered, and engaged. They are also at risk for their decision-making and that of their family, with many North American families now comprising four or five generations. The care-giver relationships are viewed by citizens of six countries on four continents as second in importance only to family relationships; more important by far then spiritual relationships, co-worker relations and financial relations. These relations are marked by compassion, understanding and partnerships and include doctors, nurses, pharmacists, other health professions, and family-based care-givers.

When health organizations in the USA have attempted to limit access of care-givers to patients or to diagnostics or therapeutics essential to the success of this relationship, they have been faced with stern rebuke. Enduring relationships in societies resist separation and respond aggressively to threats to the involved parties. The contributions of these caring relationships extend beyond day-to-day diagnostics and therapeutics. On a macro-level they are major societal stabilizers encouraging family connectiveness, absorbing and processing a populace's daily fears and worries, and generating a reservoir of trust and confidence in the future that favours investment and productivity.

The Internet is a contributing factor, as a critical technologic advance that has ended the age of information segregation. The general public is rapidly absorbing the scientific lexicon, a basic knowledge of organ function, and regularly updated theories regarding causes, diagnosis and treatment of diseases. Patients are pursuing their own research, double-checking facts, and connecting with other patients with similar conditions. Those few physicians who have created nurse-led virtual education teams have found rapid enrollment of their patients, seeking knowledge, guidance, emotional support and encouragement.

As third-generation home health managers gain knowledge and confidence caring for fourth- and fifth-generation family members, they are slowly realizing that the strategies and tactics mastered could apply equally well downstream to the benefit of themselves and the first, second and third generations.

Limited time and space in the doctor's surgery for care

A complementary factor is there is minimal time and space left in the doctor's offices for care.

The evolution of the empowered consumer care-giver is going to force change in the traditional structure of our hospital and office-based health care system. This traditional system, which need not and cannot withstand the sheer numbers of our aging population, will quietly accede to the care-giver and consumer wishes to radiate holistic care from the home. There are not the numbers of trained physicians, specialists or hospital beds to manage the capacity demands of a sick and aging society. When it comes to health care, societies must choose to stay well and to stay home.

Why does this make sense? Well first, home is where education, behavioural modification, prevention, wellness and (in the future) most early diagnosis and treatment will occur. Second, home is a more convenient and safe care site for common conditions than a hospital or clinic. Third, family care-givers will function, in the future, as part of the physician care team, and will be linked by the information highway to their doctors and nurses, and will be financially rewarded for managing their family's care.

What might the future look like under such a scenario? In the future, the physician team capacity has grown, as most care does not require a personal visit from a doctor. Physician reimbursement has increased in acknowledgement of their roles in managing clinical and education teams and multi-generational complexity. Nursing school enrollment is up; their critical role as educational director of home health manager networks is a major magnet for their profession. Health Care Teams will coordinate both clinical and educational continuums under physician oversight; most educational leadership will be delegated by physicians to nurses who will maintain 24/7 contact with Home Health Managers through Virtual Health Networks. What does this mean? Properly supported and validated by the doctor with education, behavioural modification, early diagnosis and screening, most care decisions and care functions can take place in the home. Such support has led to evolution of informal care-givers into designated Home Health Managers and their fully validated inclusion into the physician-led, nurse-managed Health Care Team.

End of life care

Does such a transformative vision for health care come out of nowhere? Is it realistic? How would it be funded?

These are all legitimate questions. To begin with, we are not starting from scratch. Let's take for example the progress that has been made in the area of end of life care, and the emergence of hospice and palliative care, increasingly an option for citizens.

If one wishes to transform health care, a good place to begin is with the examination of the dying process. It is here that you will find the challenges of multi-generational complexity, humanity, fear, dynamic belief systems, cultural influencers, and a pressing need to individualize care and manage disorganization.

MY FAMILY

In 2005, I experienced two deaths in my family. One, my 50-year-old brother-in-law, married to my younger sister – together the parents of three teenage children. The other, my wife's mother, with multiple chronic diseases and dementia, who died in her 90th year.

Both deaths involved the complexity of large family dynamics – I am one of 12 children and my wife is one of 10. Both loved ones died at home. Both had the assistance of a hospice. And both progressed through a series of stages that taxed the families' management and organizational skills.

Author and psychiatrist Elisabeth Kübler Ross described the five stages of grief as denial, anger, bargaining, depression and acceptance (Kübler Ross 2005). Roberta Temes' book, *Living with an Empty Chair*, outlines three stages – numbness, disorganization and reorganization (Cancer Survivors 2005). While both have merit, and our families encountered all eight of these stages in varying orders and in differing ways, they do not cover the more predictable organizational stages we encountered, nor do they define the management challenges associated with each stage.

Therefore I have put together what I describe as the four organizational stages of dying:

- engagement
- release
- testimony, and
- recovery.

Engagement

The first stage, engagement, focuses on confronting the threat, exploring options for combating it, making decisions about how best to proceed, and following through on those decisions. Depending on the threat, time may or may not be an issue. For my brother-in-law, facing an aggressive cancer, time was of the essence. For my mother-in-law, with diabetes and dementia, not so much.

During engagement, the patient, family and care team are expected to explore all curative options, provide clear and honest communications, invite family input, provide best recommendations, and ultimately affirm and support the patient's decision. This requires an organizational linkage that may be as uncomplicated as a trusted physician's office, as in my mother-in-law's case, or as complex as dealing with experimental research protocols and interdisciplinary cancer centers, as in my brother-in-law's case. In general, however, engagement translates into five management challenges:

1. fact finding through personal research and outreach and through expert opinion and advice, facilitated by the establishment of trust and confidence

2. decision-making, directed at type and course of therapy

3. intervention, executing on the treatment plan, whether long term or short term

4. monitoring to assess success and be able to make informed adjustments to the treatment plan, and

5. active, ongoing reassessment with focus on risks and benefits of each decision point, and consideration not only of life but also quality of life.

Release

My second stage is release. Having engaged and pursued reasonable steps to survive, without success, those involved have to acknowledge that death must now be accepted as a near-term reality. For my brother-in-law, this reality set in during a third round of chemotherapy, after two previous regimens had failed, and bowel obstruction set in during the fifth of his six months of life following diagnosis. For my mother-in-law, this was a much more subtle and personal transition. She seemed to know when the time was right, almost 'choosing her time,' and death came ten days later.

Whether chronic or acute, young or old, when a diagnosis is first made, everyone's focus is on life preservation. But a sharp decline, results of diagnostic studies, loss of control of activities of daily living, or an internal awareness can signal a transition and lead patients and families to recognize that death is approaching. Hopefulness thus collides with truthfulness. And the truth can be harsh and undeniable, especially for the young who haven't had as much time to mentally prepare. But for all ages, stage two, release, requires acceptance by both the patient and loved ones. Readiness varies, and for progress to occur, there must be alignment and a common vision of what is to come. The focus shifts from life preservation to life enhancement. Quality of remaining life is tied to adjustments in the physical environment (such as moving a bed to the ground floor) and ensuring that pain and other symptoms, such as nausea, are effectively managed. Support must be enlisted and resources marshalled.

For my brother-in-law, this meant having one of our sisters, who is a registered nurse, move in for the last two weeks of his life, working in tandem with my sister and her husband and their children. They also involved the hospice and home visits by his doctors. For my mother-in-law, during the last week, it meant that my wife's four sisters joined her and the in-house care-giver who had managed her dementia for many years. They involved the hospice to help with pain management and provide support as they accepted the dying process.

Because of the environment, we, as the family, were organized, and because the patients were relatively pain-free but fully conscious, they were able to conduct extensive and enlightened visitations during the closing days. This prepared the families and loved ones for the future and allowed what 'needed to be said' to be said. It also created a transcendent atmosphere of great spirit to mix with the seemingly unbearable sorrow and loss. Words were exchanged that we will long remember.

Testimony

With death, we arrive at the third stage: testimony. How should loved ones be remembered? This is under the control of the living. The obituary, funeral arrangements, family travel, eulogy, burial, and various memorial rituals all require attention. Of the four organizational stages of death, this may be the one most routinely mismanaged. It is critically important, not only in communicating the value and meaning of one's life, and the lives he or she touched, but also in beginning the healing process, and often allowing old wounds to be repaired, and disrupted lives to begin anew. Among the management challenges:

1. First and foremost is inclusion – involvement of as many family members and loved ones as possible.

2. Second is planning, including finances, timing of services, and communication before, during and after the ceremony.

3. Third is performance – readings, eulogies, informal story telling, photo boards, and displays of items important to the individual and the bereaved.

4. Fourth is comforting – coming together to manage those stricken, injured, and weakened by the course of events.

5. The fifth management challenge is the act of memorializing, which is an opportunity to reinforce goodness, humour, and values that deserve a spotlight. By memorializing, we challenge ourselves to live a better and more complete life.

Recovery

The final organizational stage of dying is recovery – assisting loved ones in absorbing the loss and remembering in a way that advances the physical, mental and spiritual health of the bereaved (Prigerson and Jacobs 2001). There is not a perfect path or consistent timetable, but the management challenges associated with recovery are somewhat predictable. They include managing shock, confusion and disorientation; accepting the loss; sustaining individual self-worth; pacing recovery; identifying complicated grief if it persists and seeking professional help if it's needed; and, finally, reinvesting in relationships.

STAGES OF THE DYING PROCESS

Each of these four stages of the dying process has elements in common. But each is a unique management challenge in its own right. Similarities include that each stage is complex, requires planning, demands decisions, causes fatigue, and requires team support. That said, true success comes with the insight that each of the four stages is fundamentally different – they involve different missions, players, organizational interfaces, support staff, time pressures, and measures of success.

As Elisabeth Kübler Ross said, 'For those who seek to understand it, death is a highly creative force' (Kübler Ross 2005). And this is true, but I would add that absent the ability to manage the complexity of dying, pain for all involved may be amplified, and understanding can easily slip through the cracks. And if this is true for death and dying, it is equally true for living and thriving as well.

The financial stakes

The financial stakes are high and must evolve to include more rational approaches to public, private and family investment.

In moving from intervention to prevention, late diagnosis to early diagnosis, hospital and clinic based care to home based care, and three generation families to four and five generation families, it is fair to ask, 'Who will pay?'

With the increase in patients comes a predictable increase in costs. Some of those costs are very visible and tractable. In the USA for example, it is projected that direct costs to Medicare for Alzheimer's will increase 54 per cent to 49 billion in 2010. Medicaid, which carries the burden of nursing home payments, is expected to expend 33 billion by 2010 for Alzheimer's patients, an 80 per cent increase (Prigerson 2003).

As family members critically assess the financial consequences of these difficult decisions, costs are being assigned to each option. The ability to live independently at home is less expensive than institutionalization. But, as Gail Hunt, Executive Director of The National Alliance for Care-giving, says, 'There's a reason for that. The quality of life at home is better, yes, but only the Federal Government saves money. And that's because family care-givers are the unpaid extensions of the healthcare system' (Hunt 2003). In 1992 it was roughly five times more expensive to be elderly and dependent in a nursing home versus independent in one's own home. The nursing home charge then averaged $29,000 per year. Today, the cost approaches $60,000 per year (Agency for Health Care Policy and Research [AHCPR] 1999).

Home health infrastructure is growing. Home health care covers an increasingly important constellation of health services being delivered in a patient's home setting. Under this banner exists a complex array of professional, diagnostic, and equipment-support entities that together have, with some success, kept the frail and disabled out of hospitals and out of nursing homes (Levine and Barry 2003).

- Professional services include those of doctors, nurses, dentists, dieticians, rehabilitation therapists, social workers, psychologists, podiatrists and home health aids.

- Diagnostic services include phlebotomy, ECG, Holter Monitors, Doppler testing, oximetry, radiographic studies and a variety of point-of-care tests.

- Equipment support includes IV infusion sets, ventilators and oxygen, dialysis, medical alert devices, hospital beds, wheelchairs, commodes and lifts.

The size and complexity of the investment reflects the enormity of the challenge and the multiple benefits that accrue to home-based health solutions. A surprisingly large portion of the American public is home-based or home-bound, and the numbers are rising. In America, four- and five-generation families are now commonplace; and third-generation Americans, voluntarily or involuntarily, have become the backbone of the unpaid family care-giver movement (Census 2000).

Home-based care continues to grow. It is clearly favoured by patients and families, and has well-defined benefits. They include improved patient satisfaction compared to nursing homes or hospitals; more accurate information transfer, including medical diagnosis, social assessments, and medication lists; five to seven per cent fewer medication errors; and a 22 to 26 per cent decline in acute hospitalization (Ramsdell, Swart, Jackson et al. 1989).

Who is paying for home care, since the largest portion of the care is largely unfunded? The short-term answer is America's families – contributing not only their money, but also blood, sweat, and tears. Fully 25 per cent of all US citizens are unpaid home care providers. Their contributions are critical to maintaining frail and disabled patients in home settings. In fact, their contributions, translated into dollars, exceed real dollars spent by 600 per cent. And for their good works, they are repaid in poorer personal health outcomes, depression and social isolation (Donelan, Hill, Hoffman et al. 2002).

Private technology investment

Private technology investment is a quiet, but growing support.

Home-based care-givers need inclusion and support within care teams. If we wish to use this approach long term, support for family care-givers must include financial, logistical, and emotional expenditures to stabilize what is currently, at best, an overstressed and overburdened voluntary work force.

This support will come in many forms, including private technology investment in home health (well underway today below the radar screen) to outfit homes with pervasive motion/location sensors, intelligence analytic software, personalized prompter coaching interfaces, and Internet data transfer to care networks, functionally bringing the virtual care teams and their resources into the home and obviating the need for most office visits and the vast majority of hospitalizations.

In the future, the home itself will look quite different – it will generally be more stable, productive, and controlled. Technology, originally directed at seniors with cognitive decline, cancer, and cardiovascular disease who wanted to age in place, will be advancing the health of all ages. The infrastructure for maintaining home-based wellness will include wireless sensors that track movement of people and objects in-home; intelligent software that will analyse data and provide appropriate behavioural clues and guidance; friendly, communicative interfaces through a wide range of devices, such as wristwatches, telephones, and televisions; and Internet connectivity with the rest of the health care team (Dishman 2004).

This could become our reality, but the pieces must fall into place. According to David Tennenhouse, Vice President and Director of Intel Research:

> The real challenge for research now is to explore the implications and issues associated with having hundreds of networked computers per person. These networked computers will work together to learn our habits and patterns and be proactive in providing us with the information and services we need for a healthier, safer, more productive and enjoyable life. (Dishman 2004, p.38)

In the near future, such systems could adjust behaviour in physical fitness, nutrition, social activity, and cognitive engagement. They could assist seniors with incontinence, in regular toileting, and assure better adherence to medication regimens. They could provide early diagnostics, streaming data daily to the physician-directed, nurse-led educational team, and adjust daily treatment regimens, substantially decreasing the need for on-site office visits or hospitalization (Dishman 2004).

Return to home-centered health

Voices once again are rising in the name of health care reform. The various power bases remain much as they were in 1980 – locked in position, facing year-to-year battles for funding support from public and private sources. While they have not changed, the health care world certainly has. We are now immersed in a full-blown health consumer empowerment movement in response to aging demographics, a care-giver revolution, advances in information technology, debates over risks and benefits of various treatments and therapies, and an outpatient office-based delivery system that lacks time and space to advance prevention and wellness.

In the middle of all this noise, quietly below the radar screen, health care is preparing to restructure itself from the inside out. At the end of this silent evolution, we will have a home-centered health care system that will radically realign the current players and power bases. The new system will tilt rewards to those who play prevention, and play it well (Cohen 2003).

In the future, health insurance will expand, be portable and involve multi-year commitments. They will reimburse physicians fairly for team management and incentivize home health managers by providing lower premiums to families who effectively deliver measurably positive health outcomes and effective prevention and screening. Pharmaceutical and device companies will invest in consumer education and behavioural modification, early diagnosis and prevention, and a new business model built around home-centric health solutions. Health information highways will be home-centric; that is begin in the home, extend out to the care-givers and loop back to the home, rather than the other way around.

At the center of this home-centered health scenario will be the American family – aging in place, now routinely four- and five-generations deep, rather than just three. Family care-givers, currently present in 25 per cent of American families, are providing most of the care for parents and grandparents (Alliance for Aging Research 2002). In the next decade, they will embrace the designated role of home health manager and apply their skills up and down the generational divide as designated members of physicians' health care teams (Magee 2001).

Those teams will carry out both educational and clinical missions. The educational support teams will be coordinated with the physicians' active support, primarily by nurse educators connected 24/7 to virtual networks of family-based home health managers. Through this network, home health managers will receive targeted education, behavioural modification strategies, and financial rewards in the form of reduced insurance premiums for achieving superior outcomes for family members. Physicians, as well, will be tied to performance and fairly reimbursed for team management responsibilities (Nash 2001).

Why might this version be right?

1. There is inadequate funding, time, and space to manage an aging, actively disease-ridden population.

2. Education, behavioural modification, and preventive screening must be home-based to be successful.

3. The complexity of a four- and five-generation family becomes rapidly unmanageable in the absence of active health planning.

4. Success in managing home-based health prevention saves time and money, in the short and long term.

5. Most people don't want to go to a hospital unless they absolutely have to.

Summary

A home-centered health care system, where information begins at home, connects to physicians and care teams, and circles back home, seems impossible only because the pieces of our system, built long ago for vertical disease intervention, are locked in place by historic silos and outdated business plans. But we are now moving toward a horizontal model of health care, one that flattens the old silos, rearranges and reconstructs the pieces, and connects all the players together in a much more logical way. In the future, if you are not on the inside of this model, you will most assuredly be left out.

At the end of the day, caring will re-center in the home where caring, compassion and personalization reside. Here caring will integrate mind, body and spirit; bring together faith values and science; focus on wellness and functionality; integrate and prioritize resources along the four or five generation family divide; and tailor care to the unique cultural, social and spiritual needs of family members.

Homes will look to their communities for value grounding, integrated social systems, and resources by exclusion if overwhelmed by complexity. Physicians and nurses will advocate for these changes because they make sense and are the only reasonable way to manage the cost and quality demands of global aging societies.

This process and this more personalized care at home could facilitate the 'learning to grow old' in the way that Paul Tournier described in his book by that name. Interestingly it will have been scientific technological advances that have made this possible and that have assisted us to value more highly the wisdom of the elderly and their various faith perspectives.

References

Administration Association for Homes and Services for the Aging (AAHSA) (1999) 'Nursing homes' [fact sheet]. Available at: www.aahsa.org/public/nursbkg.htm. Accessed 16 June 1999.

Agency for Health Care Policy and Research (AHCPR) (1999) 'Research on long-term care expenditures for healthcare.' Available at: www.ahcpr.gov/research/longtrm1.htm. Accessed 30 August 1999.

Alliance for Aging Research (2002) *Medical Never-Never Land: Ten Reasons Why America is Not Ready for the Coming Age Boom*. Washington, D.C.: AAR Available at: www.agingresearch.org/brochures/nevernever/nevernever.pdf. Accessed 26 June 2006.

Bishop, C.E. (1999) 'Where are the missing elders? The decline in nursing home use, 1985 and 1995.' *Health Aff 18*, 146–155.

Cancer Survivors (2005) 'Cancer Survivors Online.' Available at: www.cancersurvivors.org/Coping/end%20term/stages.htm. Accessed 19 May.

Census 2000 Brief. 'The 65 years and over population: 2000.' Available at: http://www.census.gov/prod/2001/pubs/c2kbr01-10.pdf. Accessed 25 July 2003.

Cohen, J.L. (2003) 'Human population: The next half century.' *Science 302*, 1172–1175.

Dishman, E. (2004) 'Inventing wellness systems for aging in place.' *Computer 37*, 34–41.

Donelan K., Hill C.A., Hoffman C., Scoles, K. et al. (2002) 'Challenged to care: informal care-givers in a changing health system.' *Health Aff (Millwood) 21*, 222–231.

Havens, B. (1990) *Improving the Health of Older People. A World View.* Oxford: Oxford University Press.

Hunt, G. (2003) 'Aging – Part 3: New Environments for Mature Living.' *Health Politics,* 20 August.

Kübler Ross, E. (2005) Available at: www.elisabethkublerross.com. Accessed 19 May 2005.

Levine, S.A. and Barry, P.P. (2003) 'Home care.' In C.K. Cassel, R.M. Leipzig, H.J. Cohen, E.B. Larson et al. (eds) *Geriatric Medicine: An Evidence-Based Approach,* 4th edn. New York, NY: Springer-Verlag.

Magee, M. (2001) *The Best Medicine.* New York: St Martin's Press.

MetLife and National Alliance for Care-giving (2004) *Miles Away: The MetLife Study of Long-Distance Care-giving.'* Westport, CT: MetLife Mature Market Institute. Available at: www.caregiving.org/ data/milesaway.pdf. Accessed 26 June 2006.

Nash, D. (2001) *Connecting with the New Health Care Consumer.* New York: McGraw-Hill.

Nostrand, J.F. van, Clark, R.F. and Romoren, T.I. (1993) 'Long-term care use by the elderly: Nursing home care in five nations.' *Ageing Int 20,* 2, 1–5.

Ory, M.G., Hoffman, R.R., Yee, J.L., Tennstedt, S. and Schulz, R. (1999) 'Prevalence and impact of care-giving: a detailed comparison between dementia and non-dementia care-givers.' *Gerontologist 39,* 177–185.

Perls, T.T. (1997) 'Centarians prove the compression of morbidity hypothesis, but what about the rest of us who are genetically less fortunate?' *Med Hypotheses 49,* 405–407.

Prigerson, H.G. (2003) 'Costs to society of family care-giving for patients with end stage Alzheimer's disease.' *NEJM 349,* 1891–1892.

Prigerson, H.G. and Jacobs, S.C. (2001) 'Caring for bereaved patients: all the doctors just suddenly go.' *JAMA 286,* 1369–1376.

Ramsdell, J.W., Swart, J.A., Jackson, J.E., Renwall, M. *et al.* (1989) 'The yield of home visits in the assessment of geriatric patients.' *J Am Geriatr Soc 37,* 17–24.

Schultz, R., Mendelsohn, A.B., Haley, W.E., Mahoney, D. *et al.* (2003) 'End-of-life care and the effects of bereavement on family care-givers of persons with dementia.' *NEJM 349,* 1936–1942.

Shalala, D. (1999) 'The United States Special Committee on Aging. Long Term Care for the Twenty-First Century: A Common Sense Proposal to Support Family Care-givers.' Testimony before the United States Special Committee on Aging. Available at: www.senate.gov/~aging/hr29.htm. Accessed 4 October.

CHAPTER 14
NEUROSCIENCE AND BELIEF: A CHRISTIAN PERSPECTIVE

Andrew Sims

Introduction

At first sight it is difficult to see how there could be any conflict between science and belief; after all, they seem to belong to different realms. Historically, however, there has been mutual antagonism; sometimes quite unnecessary and based on misunderstandings, sometimes deliberately confrontational. This chapter is written by a Christian psychiatrist, who uses the findings of neuroscience in his practice, but also sees the relevance of Christian belief to his medical work, just as Paul Tournier brought insights gained from the Bible and his life experience as a Christian to his practice as a physician in Switzerland (Tournier 1954). The Christian living in the twenty-first century does not inhabit two different worlds. Much more, he or she lives in one world with myriad, sometimes conflicting ideologies. Just after the Second World War Tournier wrote about all conflictual situations in *The Strong and the Weak*:

> Only religious faith can supply the calm, creative strength which, far from strengthening one man at another's expense, is propagated from one to the other. 'It is many years now,' writes one of my brother doctors, 'since I acquired the "technique" of our profession...but long ago I learnt that it does not work without faith...the whole of psychology is useless if men are not rooted in a sound conception of life'. (Tournier 1947, p.238)

This chapter explores this connection between faith and practice in the field of mental health and illness, looking first at the nature of neuroscience and then relating this to significant issues for belief such as cause and effect, free will, and the effects of religion on health. This leads to a concluding section discussing some basic Christian theological themes, such as the nature of God as love, the believer's experience of 'being in Christ' and harmony with God and in the world.

What is neuroscience?

Neuroscience is 'the study of the brain' (Ramachandran 2003). If the abstraction we normally refer to as 'the mind' has any location, then that must be in the brain. So, the neurosciences are closely concerned with the function and topography of human behaviour and emotion, and their disorders.

The basic sciences of physics, chemistry and biology, when applied to the brain and its functions, have spawned several separate scientific disciplines. These have in common their use of the scientific method of formulation of hypotheses, with experiments directed at testing these and replication. *The New Oxford Textbook of Psychiatry* recognizes ten separate areas of current interest for the neuroscientific basis of psychiatric disorders (Gelder, López-Ibor and Andreasen 2000). *Neuroanatomy* is concerned with the topographical organization of the brain and spinal cord, and the anatomical connections forming functional pathways in the central nervous system (CNS). *Neurodevelopment* charts the origins of the CNS from specialized ectoderm through to the development of the brain and the detailed anatomy of the cerebral cortices.

Neuroendocrinology is concerned with the chemistry linking different parts of the brain, especially the hypothalamus and the pituitary, with other parts of the body, for example, thyroid, adrenals, gonads and mammary gland. *Neurotransmitters* are chemicals released into the body and having an effect on specific receptors in different parts of the brain. There are Class 1 neuroreceptors that react to the neurotransmitters within milliseconds, and slower acting, Class 2 receptors, which modulate signals generated by Class 1 receptors.

Formerly, *neuropathology* concentrated upon obvious lesions of the brain such as tumour, infection, vascular disease, trauma, toxic and hypoxic conditions, and degenerative brain diseases. Now much greater pathophysiological sophistication is possible with *positron emission tomography* (PET) and *single-photon emission tomography* (SPET). *Magnetic resonance imaging* (MRI) is a technique, which is developing all the time, for visualizing the structure, function and metabolism of the living human brain. It has the great advantage of making visual and clear contrast between grey matter, white matter and cerebrospinal fluid. Functional MRI is particularly useful for measuring changes in cerebral blood flow, which follow changes in brain activity.

Two other human biological, scientific disciplines are also very important in understanding the working of the human brain. These are *psycho-neuroimmunology*, concerned with interactions between brain and the immune system and their clinical implications, and *genetics*.

A significant contribution to the understanding of many psychiatric disorders is made by *genetics*. For some conditions, such as Huntington's chorea and acute intermittent porphyria, which both have autosomal dominant inheritance, there can be no understanding of the condition without taking genetics into account. In several mental disorders, for example schizophrenia, family, twin and adoption studies provide significant information about the condition. Gene mapping is now being applied to major psychiatric illnesses and molecular genetics is already having an effect upon psychiatric nosology (Craddock and Owen 2005).

As well as the disciplines derived from basic sciences described above, *experimental psychology* and *epidemiology* both make important contributions to neuroscientific understanding. In psychiatry, psychological theory often forms the spring board for testable hypotheses using neuroscientific technology. Also, psychology provides measuring tools where there are no appropriate physical parameters. With increased sophistication of both demonstrating the physical substrates for mental activity and psychological measurement, an understanding of the physical basis of psychopathology becomes increasingly possible (Liddle 2001). Epidemiology, the study of numbers of people presenting any particular characteristic in a defined human population, is essential for understanding the results, and differences demonstrated, of scientific measurement.

Neuroscience and religion – conflict or complementarity?

There is a history of unproductive conflict between science and religious belief. Those of us who are now practising or applying a scientific discipline and also hold religious beliefs have inherited a battlefield from our predecessors – and many unexploded mines are still left there for the unwary. Although many of the great discoverers, such as Galileo, saw every detail of the universe as yet further evidence of the hand of God in creation, in the late nineteenth and first two-thirds of the twentieth centuries, many academic scientists were aligned with atheism, and so science and religious faith became polarized, with the latter often regarded as obscurantist.

It is helpful at this point to see science in three guises, to the ordinary person: science as fact; science as hypothesis; and science as dogma. The detailed work and progress made in different neuroscientific disciplines, as described in the last section, are an example of science as fact. Each piece of new knowledge is achieved by application of scientific method, and gradually more is known about increasingly sophisticated functions of the brain. It is hoped that these findings can be used for the intelligent treatment of patients with specific disorders. Whatever their belief system, mental health professional staff and patients alike will undoubtedly welcome this.

Science has progressed by forming hypotheses, which are *falsifiable*; that is, the notion is stated in such quantifiable terms that an experiment can be carried out to disprove the hypothesis if it is incorrect. This is how further discoveries are made and, even though most hypotheses may prove fallacious, this process is essential for progress. At any time there are many hypotheses in the neurosciences awaiting further experiment. As an example, the maternal–foetal origins hypothesis suggests that exposure of the foetus to an adverse environment in utero leads to permanent programming of tissue function and subsequent increased risk of developing adult cardiovascular and metabolic diseases (Barker 1998).

It is important that we know what is established fact and what is hypothesis, and that the two do not become blurred because of the enthusiasm of the individual scientist, the strength of his or her convictions or the authority he or she carries because of past work or recognition. Neuroscience has a tendency towards simplistic reductionism, and the possibility of ever linking mental processes to precise brain location has been challenged (Uttal 2001). High-level cognitive processes are associated with widely distributed activity in many parts of the brain and there are doubts about the definitions of those processes themselves.

Much science teaching, both at school and undergraduate level, is given dogmatically. Laws of physics and chemical formulae are learnt by rote. Ridicule may be cast on those who ask questions. It is quite possible that the current unpopularity of science at undergraduate level is partly due to the dilemma with which students are presented: advances come through exploring original hypotheses but these can only be produced after the humdrum business of learning a mass of facts. Most students never get beyond this stage – it is all remembering laws and formulae. Those who believe in God have a particular problem with the scientific dogma of randomness. As every statistician knows, randomness is quite difficult to achieve. Nothing in the natural world happens by chance. The concept is untenable to anyone, such as a doctor, trying to solve problems by logical steps.

Both theists and atheists have a problem with the balance between determinism and free will, for differing reasons.

A refutation of randomness is needed for psychiatric practice. Rational treatment is based upon a diagnostic formulation in psychiatry, and for this descriptive psychopathology, including observation of the patient and empathic understanding of the subjective state, is crucial. If human behaviour or thought processes were seen to be random, then thinking itself and the speech resulting from it becomes meaningless, mere epiphenomena of the underlying chemical mechanisms. For the Christian a belief in randomness as the ultimate motivating force is incompatible with the omnipotence and omnipresence of God. One cannot discuss science and belief without alluding to this dilemma over causes.

Cause and effect

On the one hand science is orderly, it conforms to 'rules' and to a basic pattern of cause and effect. On the other hand, some claim that it has evolved by a series of random processes, all due to chance. These two notions are ultimately irreconcilable, and fly in the face of common sense. Dogma has emerged from hypothesis without the inconvenience of proof.

Science and faith are agreed that all that goes on in the world, the universe, the micro-organism, is explicable by cause and effect. This is true of the physical world in the 'laws' of physics and chemistry. It is also true for human cognition and behaviour; as psychiatrists we can only function within the basic premise that all behaviour is ultimately understandable and meaningful, at least for the person who carries out that behaviour at the time he does so (Jaspers 1959; Sims 2003). This is so fundamental for human relationships that it is normally taken for granted. Behaviour (including thinking behaviour) is never random, not an epiphenomenon, but always reflects the basic principle of cause and effect. The biological psychiatrist will be looking for chemical, genetic or structural causes of her patient's depressive illness, and acting accordingly in terms of treatment. The psychotherapist will be seeking the roots of motivation for dysfunctional patterns of behaviour in adverse experiences in childhood or earlier. Both assume as a *sine qua non* for their practice that the principle of cause and effect is operating.

Randomness is merely a statement of ignorance, never an adequate explanation. It is an abstraction, a 'let us assume' of science. It imposes the rules of the group to subsume the specific forces upon the individual. So, one takes a coin and tosses it 100 times. In this series, the coin comes down 50 times as 'heads' and 50 as 'tails'. A random process, or is it? For the captain who tosses and shouts, each action is random, but not for the ultimately equipped physicist. If one knows every single force upon that coin at every point of the toss and fall, then one can predict the outcome with 100 per cent certainty. *Chance* was merely an expression of ignorance.

Nothing we know about in the natural world happens by chance; the more we know about it the more we know about its logical causation. When a doctor talks about 'random mutation' of a gene or 10 per cent mortality with an operation, she or he is giving risks in statistical terms. If all the factors for this individual having this operation were known – the patient, the surgeon, the hospital, and so on – then one could predict likely outcome with great accuracy. *Random mutation*, in the individual case, is also an expression of ignorance concerning the precise influences at work on the chromosome.

Similarly, there are no 'random' thoughts, feelings, motivation, behaviour or even psychiatric disorders. The sister of a person diagnosed as suffering from schizophrenia learns that she has a 16 per cent lifetime risk of developing the condition herself. The more we know about the patient, the sister, the diagnostic criteria used, the social background, and so on, the more accurate we can be in giving a prognosis for her.

The words shouted by a person with a long-term schizophrenic illness sitting on a park bench are never meaningless, arbitrary or random. They have meaning, at least for the person himself at the time he utters them. Randomness is not an adequate theory for what cannot otherwise be explained. We are left with a paradox, shared by science and religion.

Determinism versus free will

Issues of causality come to a head when we consider human behaviour, whether in its 'normal' or its pathological forms. Here we encounter the perennial debate about determinism versus free will. I shall not try to give a full account of it here, but instead consider the key topic of addiction as an illustration of the problem. I suggest that, in practice, clinicians work upon an assumption of free will, even though it is obvious that this is often severely compromised. Insights from the Christian doctrines of sin and redemption can shed light on this complexity.

Let us take as an example altered states of consciousness due to drugs or brain assault, and limits to freedom imposed by social and cultural background. Having drunk ten pints of beer shortly before committing a felony is unlikely to be accepted as mitigation, although it may be an explanation. The father and uncles of the accused having served prison sentences for a similar offence is also unlikely to conjure leniency from the magistrates.

Christians are used to grappling with this concept because of belief in the doctrine of sin, without which redemption is unnecessary and impossible. Sin can be regarded both as an act and a tendency. This is an important topic for human behaviour and behavioural medicine. There are analogies here with addiction, and Cook (2005) has drawn helpful parallels: members of Alcoholics Anonymous do not regard themselves as being 'mad', in the sense of suffering from psychotic disorder, or even a neurotic or personality disorder. They have a sense of addictive disorders as standing apart, in a category of their own and to be treated within a framework of rational discourse and personal responsibility. Whereas informed professionals and organizations, such as AA, consider such people to be sufferers from a disease, wider society has usually seen addicts as being 'bad', the source of their own troubles. To quote Cook:

> the addictions paradigm is a useful model to assist theology in its understanding of sin. It reveals much more clearly than is often apparent that the spiritual issue of sin is inseparable from the psychological and biological experiences of human life… On a daily basis, we all experience a range of different desires, which compete with each other more or less successfully. Some we indulge and others we don't. Some we indulge occasionally, and others regularly. Some we become rather attached to – or perhaps addicted to. (Cook 2005)

The notion of the 'divided will' has been developed by St Paul: 'For I do not do the good I want, but the evil I do not want is what I do' (Rom 7:19, New Revised Standard Version), and also St Augustine: 'And so I was at war with myself and torn apart by myself. And this strife was against my will' (Pine-Coffin 1961). The phenomenological experience of the addict is similar to the experience of anyone who has found themself subjectively drawn toward engaging in behaviour that they believe to be morally wrong. The more often the alcoholic 'gives in', the more difficult does it become not to drink next time, and, mercifully, vice versa.

A Christian outlook in this area can contribute to understanding and potential 'treatment' of the problem. The absolutist approach of the media, whereby if a celebrity transgresses in his twenties he is damned for the rest of his life, is unhelpful. So is the denial of any morality, good or evil, by extreme libertarians. The Christian accepts that wrong-doing not only happens but is universal; it can enslave and become habitual. But forgiveness, reconciliation and restitution are also possible and there is always hope for the person who has failed to achieve their own standard and regrets it. This forgiveness continues. The sinner sins again, the alcoholic drinks again; forgiveness, restitution always remains possible.

This is also linked to our response of *repentance* – changing our minds. The media gives the impression that there can be no change of heart; once a serial rapist, always such, for example. Belief in a merciful God allows King David, after rape and murder, to write:

> For I know my transgressions,
> and my sin is always before me...
> Create in me a pure heart, O God,
> and renew a steadfast spirit within me.
> Psalm 51:3,10. (New International Version 1973)

The believer is assured that *forgiveness,* a change of heart and a change of direction is possible through God's act of redemption.

For some time, it has been thought that some people may have a biological sensitivity to develop alcohol misuse. This has been investigated with biochemical and neurophysiological markers and using molecular genetics (Negrete 2000). Also, it has been known that alcohol misuse is transmitted through families, both genetically and socially. There is an increase above expected of both alcohol abusers and teetotalers in the families of alcoholics. Does this mean that such individuals have no freedom of action, entirely at the whim of their brain chemistry and genes?

No, unlike Huntington's chorea in which genetics predicts the occurrence of the condition independent of other factors, the inheritance for alcoholism is of a *tendency*. On each occasion the individual decides for himself whether he will have another drink or not. In each drinking bout, after each drink, the decision not to drink again becomes more difficult, and after each bout, the decision not to start another also becomes harder. But there is still an element of choice, and treatment, or help, is directed towards strengthening that resolve not to drink again on the next and every future occasion.

The effects of religion on health

It is only 40 years since the standard British textbook of psychiatry stated that religion is for 'the hesitant, the guilt-ridden, the excessively timid, those lacking clear convictions with which to face life' (Mayer-Gross, Slater and Roth 1954, 1960 and 1969, p.180). Religion was regarded both as a symptom of mental illness caused, on occasions, by religious experience, and bad for your health in terms of outcome. Psychiatrists holding religious beliefs were regarded as being seriously unscientific.

But was this a reasoned view or a prejudice? Science is prediction. The hypothesis states that, what will follow this chain of specific circumstances, is this particular outcome. Medicine is also into prediction – giving a prognosis. In psychiatry prognosis is based upon epidemiological principles. What happens, with what frequency, to a defined population with this condition in these circumstances? It is generally based upon a large sample of the population, and those selected for the sample should be representative of the whole population to be studied.

An important and intriguing question is whether religious belief can, of itself, alter prognosis. Over recent years in many studies in all areas of health and illness, religious belief and/or practice has been recorded as a variable for outcome studies, in most instances as an incidental piece of information, with no intention by the researchers of exploring it specifically. The findings of these disparate studies have been collected by Koenig, McCullough and Larson (2001) in a comprehensive monograph, which covers the whole of medicine and is based on 1200 research studies and 400 reviews. There are large sections of this book on both physical and mental illnesses; the research quality of each paper is evaluated quantitatively, and religious belief is explored using several different measures. Most of the studies come from the USA, and the religion is mostly Christian or Jewish, with few from other religions.

Overall, religious belief is associated with better health outcome for physical and mental illnesses, which is a huge claim. The authors are extremely cautious in drawing conclusions but the results are overwhelming. To quote from mental health studies:

> In the majority of studies, religious involvement is correlated with well-being, happiness and life satisfaction; hope and optimism; purpose and meaning in life; higher self-esteem; adaptation to bereavement; greater social support and less loneliness; lower rates of depression and faster recovery from depression; lower rates of suicide and fewer positive attitudes towards suicide; less anxiety; less psychosis and fewer psychotic tendencies; lower rates of alcohol and drug use and abuse; less delinquency and criminal activity; greater marital stability and satisfaction. We concluded that, for the vast majority of people, the apparent benefit of devout religious belief and practice probably outweigh the risks. (Koenig *et al.* 2001, p.228)

It is almost as if the authors themselves are surprised by their findings.

Correlations between religious belief and greater wellbeing 'typically equal or exceed correlations between wellbeing and other psychosocial variables, such as social support' (Koenig *et al.* 2001, p.215). That is a massive assertion, comprehensively attested to by a large volume of evidence. In George Brown's studies on the social origins of depression (Brown and Harris 1978) various types of social support were the most powerful protective factors against depression. Of 93 cross-sectional or prospective studies of the relationship between religious involvement and depression in Koenig *et al.* (1997), 60 (65%) reported a significant positive relationship between a measure of religious involvement and lower rates of depression; 13 studies reported no association; four reported greater depression among the more religious; and 16 studies gave mixed findings.

The authors develop a model for how and why religious belief and practice might influence mental health. There are direct beneficial effects upon mental health, such as better cognitive appraisal and coping behaviour in response to stressful life experiences. There are also indirect effects, such as developmental factors and even genetic (Egan *et al.* 1996) and biological, for example, immunological (Koenig *et al.* 1997) factors.

There are also the benefits of being within the social structure of a faith community.

These findings are perhaps not really surprising. In general, religion encourages a broadly healthy lifestyle; having a systematic set of meanings in life encourages optimism; and the Church can be a strongly supportive organization. Religious belief is a valid variable that should be taken into account by epidemiological science. However, there is no evidence to suggest that seeking religious affiliation for its potential health benefits would be successful.

Negative health consequences of religion have included failure of timely seeking of medical care and replacing medical care, inappropriately, with religion. Authoritarianism and prejudice in religion can endanger the health of individuals. However, the evidence for negative effects of religion on mental health rest largely on a few, isolated case reports.

Religion complementing science for mental health
RELATIONSHIP AS A WORLD VIEW
Science, especially chemistry, is concerned with interaction: the relationship between two or more different natures when they come together. Physics is concerned with the interplay of different forces and their consequences – electricity, mechanics, light, sound, hydrodynamics and nuclear physics. Biological studies, being concerned with the physiology of different organs working together, and the workings of each organ individually in contributing its functions, and ecology, in its study of the interaction of different organisms in the environment, show the same principle.

Cause results in effect when two or more causes come together. At the micro-level, science looks at the interaction between atoms; at the macro-level, interaction between cosmic bodies. Neuroscience is concerned with brain interactions and their behavioural manifestations. All of science is totally involved with relationship.

> The Christian view is that one of the chief goals of creation and evolution is the emergence of beings that to some extent possess awareness, creative agency, and powers of reactive and responsible relationship... (Ward 1998)

Keith Ward, in his interesting book, develops the theme that God, in every aspect of His creation, is concerned with relationship; this was a purpose of the creation of the world. Human beings are organisms of relationship; being human essentially involves relating to other humans. We can only fully develop self through relationship with others. All mental illnesses manifest a disturbance of relationship.

The human spirit gives us the possibility of relationship with God. Our relationship with each other may be more or less equal in terms of giving and receiving; it is never equal with God. He gives and we receive. What we can give back in relationship is living with each other and the world in harmony, and prayer, which is what we call our communication with God.

What if neuroscience can localize prayer, or what has been called transcendence? Does this invalidate prayer? In a PET study investigating relationships between serotonin 5-HT(1A) receptor density and personality traits, the binding potential was found to be correlated inversely with scores for self-transcendence, 'a personality trait covering religious behaviour and attitudes'. It was concluded that the serotonin system may serve as a biological marker for spiritual experiences (Borg *et al.* 2003). Could it be considered that spiritual experiences merely represent an irritation of the brain at this location? No, if this localization is correct, this indicates where it is mediated. It does not explain away its happening, or the relationship with God, any more than an analysis of the wood fibre explains away the meaning of the article in a newspaper.

GOD OF LOVE
The positive and non-destructive relationship between God and humankind is called love. From this emanates positive relationship between person and person. Such loving actions and relationships form the cement of human society, and enable that society to function successfully and harmoniously.

If we are going to bring the concept of love into medicine, we also have to introduce the notion of values. Medical values are different from moral or aesthetic values (Fulford 1989). However, when adding a spiritual element, medical, moral and aesthetic values are all relevant. Science is, by definition, without values or, in that sense, valueless. Although science itself is without values, its application, for example, in medicine, necessarily involves values. Also, the scientist will always be working to their own individual values, even if it is only to regard values as a bad thing. There is here a considerable difference in outlook that can have practical implications, certainly at the extremes. The logical outcome of a doctor regarding himself as a 'pure scientist', and therefore ignoring values, will be very different from a doctor who strives to put the value of love at the centre of his or her practice. A patient is likely to find the latter doctor 'caring' and the former 'callous'.

Of course, the English word 'love' has multiple meanings (Lewis 1960). At one end of the spectrum, love may imply a selfish and possessive domination of another; at the other end, an anaemic legalism, 'I am only doing this because I love you'. (For love read 'cannot stand you but am doing this because of moral obligation'). Neither of these describe the total love of God for us and our, when we as humans are at our best, replicating this in our relationship with each other.

Thus the affinity of atoms for other atoms, when transferred to the human arena, can be transformed into love. This is difficult to explain neuroscientifically but it is never random, always cause and effect. Hate, and consequential destruction, is a perversion of the human capacity for love; it is still based upon relationship.

In Christian belief, this love is not mere mutuality, but something that has been given to us at enormous cost. We believe that God became man in order to redeem individual human beings through the death of that man, Jesus Christ, so that each of us can be reconciled with God for ever. True love is always revealed in cost. The love of God shows itself in that it is not we who are striving to find God, but He is actively searching for us. God gives total love, including giving himself. In the words of the late Pope John Paul II: 'In the love that pours forth from the heart of Christ we find hope for the future of the world. Christ has redeemed the world: "By his wounds we are healed" (Isaiah 53:5)' (His Holiness Pope John Paul II 2005).

PERSONAL RELATIONSHIP WITH JESUS CHRIST

Those subscribing to the dogma of science, who are hostile to Christian faith, often make the mistake of launching their attacks on the traditions and ceremonies of the Church, and wondering why these are still significant in the twenty-first century. The power of faith is not in its history but in the shared belief that Christ is risen from the dead, is alive now and has become, and remains, part of *my* everyday experience.

This can neither be explained, nor repudiated, in neuroscientific terms. The notions of 'being in Christ', 'with Christ', 'Christ in me',

'Christ with me' can be explored with the methods of phenomenological psychopathology (Sims 2002).

When a believer makes such statements as these, one of two psychiatric states could be, and have been, used to explain it. In a *passivity experience* or *delusion of control*, the patient, most often suffering from schizophrenia, states that there is control of their innermost self by an outside influence. This experience is described in concrete, even physical terms; the influence is described as alien, even against the true self and its will. This abnormal experience is one type of disorder of the boundaries of self, which could be explained by specific disturbance of brain function (Sims 1993). The spiritual description by the believer is of an internal experience, of God being inside, helping, making the person more truly what they want to do and be.

The other psychiatric explanation used is what is described as *trance and possession disorder* in the International Classification of Disorders (World Health Organization 1992): a temporary loss of the individual's identity and awareness of their surroundings; occasionally the individual appears to have been taken over by another personality or 'spirit'. This description does fit occasional, ecstatic religious experiences, but the vast majority of everyday accounts from believers that God is *within* are quite different, and not associated with the altered state of consciousness that is part of possession state. Neither of these psychiatric conditions come anywhere near my ordinary experience of the indwelling presence of God.

The concept of locus of control is relevant. Personal control (or degree of perceived choice) is a strong predictor of happiness (Myers and Diener 1996). Whilst believing that God is inside and in control might appear to suggest an external locus of control, research studies have shown a significant positive relationship between religious belief and internal locus of control (Jackson and Coursey 1988). An internalized faith, with prayer, empowers the believer to change their situation and deny the tyranny of an all-powerful, external 'fate'. The spiritual belief of the presence of God is experienced as 'inside' and 'on my side', and not as an arbitrary, external and potentially destructive force.

Such ideas of being within the love of God become incorporated into the concept of self and self-image. *Amor ergo sum*: I am loved, therefore I am. My feelings of self-worth and self-confidence are predicated by my acceptance by God as being loved. We only find our personal God from a position of need, on our knees.

HARMONY: WITH GOD AND IN THE WORLD

Common to many of the philosophies emanating from scientific dogmatism is the idea of natural selection producing a progressively improved human race. Achieving status, knowing the 'secrets', is focused on the intellectually most superior. This is diametrically opposite to the teaching of Jesus: 'whoever wants to become great among you must be your servant, and whoever wants to be first must be slave of all' (Mark 10: 43–44, New International Version). Also: 'Love the Lord your God with all your heart and with all your soul and with all your mind and with all your strength.' The second is this: 'Love your neighbour as yourself' (Mark 12: 30–31 New International Version). Spirituality emanating from evolutionary theory produces competitiveness and elitism, whereas Christian teaching aims at harmony between human beings and service by the stronger for the weaker.

The quality of the relationship with God and with other people is mutually dependent. 'I tell you the truth, whatever you did for one of the least of these brothers of mine, you did for me' (Matthew 25:40, New International Version). Jesus' teaching on relationships is summarized in the parable of the Good Samaritan (Luke 10:25–37). The good neighbour to the injured man was a member of a despised race who took pity on him, gave practical care for his injuries and paid his expenses – that is, had mercy on him. This is also the theme of Tolstoy's short story about the altruistic cobbler who wanted to draw near to God ('Where Love is, God is', Tolstoy 1885).

Harmony with God is expressed in harmony with mankind. It is based on forgiveness, to be forgiven by God and to forgive other people, and reconciliation, with God and with others. Christian teaching is based upon altruism, even self-sacrifice, and rejects 'survival of the fittest' or 'the selfish gene' (Dawkins 1989). This leads to the Church being seen as a supportive community, which is one of the major reasons for religious involvement resulting in better outcome from a range of illnesses (Koenig *et al.* 2001).

This is not a problem with science itself, but some have made scientific ideas a source of spirituality. Adherents of the *selfish gene* have to go through polemical acrobatics to try and fit altruism into their schema. When we see glimmers of godly harmony, Christians regard this as a sign of the coming of the Kingdom of Heaven.

Conclusions

Neuroscience explores the form and function of the brain. It uses many different technologies to do so. It also relies on the behavioural and social sciences, and statistics applied to populations in epidemiology. A Christian doctor welcomes the findings of neuroscience and applies them avidly for the benefit of patients. Neuroscience and belief can work together and be mutually helpful and illuminating.

Problems arise when Christians are either arrogant or fearful towards the findings of science. The possibilities produced by advances in technology inevitably result in ethical dilemmas.

Sometimes scientific hypothesis has been promulgated as fact, taught as dogma, and converted, often by non-scientists, into philosophy or even religion. On occasions one scientific principle has been promoted to the exclusion of all others, and this can result in distortion. For example, if one breaks a leg the biological principles of bone healing are much more relevant than evolutionary theory.

The hypothesis of randomness runs counter to Christian thinking, especially if it is used to explain human behaviour. The dilemma of determinism and free will is a challenge for believers and non-believers alike.

Religion is a much neglected factor in studying prognosis and health outcomes. It is important to assess the effect of belief and ascertain why this should be. Relationship as a world view develops from Christian theology and is also a basis for the practice of psychiatry. The love of God is a lynch-pin of Christian belief and how this relates to neuroscience has been explored. Also the possibility of a personal relationship with Jesus Christ is essential, and how such a belief, compares with psychiatric syndromes of passivity and possession state has been discussed. Harmony, with its associations with forgiveness and reconciliation, shows valuable insights that faith can bring to medical practice.

References

Barker, D. (1998) *Mothers, Babies and Health in Later Life.* Edinburgh: Churchill Livingstone.

Borg, J., Andrée, B., Soderstrom, H. and Farde, L. (2003) 'The serotonin system and spiritual experiences.' *American Journal of Psychiatry 160,* 1965–1969.

Brown, G.W. and Harris, T.O. (1978) *Social Origins of Depression.* London: Tavistock.

Cook, C. (2005) 'Personal responsibility and Its Relationship to Substance Misuse.' In M.D. Beer and N. Pocock *'Mad or Bad?' Christian Responses to Those who do 'Antisocial' Things in the Context of Mental Disorder.* London: Hodder and Stoughton.

Craddock, N. and Owen, M.J. (2005) 'The beginning of the end for the Kraepelinian dichotomy.' *British Journal of Psychiatry 186*, 364–366.

Dawkins, R. (1989) *The Selfish Gene.* Oxford: Oxford University Press.

Egan, K.M., Newcomb, P.A., Longnecker, M.P. *et al.* (1996) 'Jewish religion and risk of breast cancer.' *Lancet 347*, 1645–1646.

Fulford, W.K.M. (1989) *Moral Theory and Medical Practice.* Cambridge: Cambridge University Press.

Gelder, M., López-Ibor, J.J. and Andreasen, N.C. (eds) (2000) *New Oxford Textbook of Psychiatry.* Oxford: Oxford University Press.

His Holiness Pope John Paul II (2005) *Memory and Identity: Personal Reflections.* London: Weidenfeld and Nicolson.

Jackson, L.E. and Coursey, R.D. (1988) 'The relationship of God control and internal locus of control to intrinsic religious motivation, coping and purpose in life.' *Journal for the Scientific Study of Religion 27*, 399–410.

Jaspers, K. (1959) *General Psychopathology,* 7th edn (transl. J. Hoenig and M.W. Hamilton, 1963). Manchester: Manchester University Press.

Koenig, H.G., Cohen, H.J., George, L.K. *et al.* (1997) 'Attendance at religious services, interleukin-6, and other biological indicators of immune function in older adults.' *International Journal of Psychiatry in Medicine 27*, 233–250.

Koenig, H.G., McCullough, M.E. and Larson, D.B. (2001) *Handbook of Religion and Health.* Oxford: Oxford University Press.

Lewis, C.S. (1960) *The Four Loves.* London: Harper Collins.

Liddle, P.F. (2001) *Disordered Mind and Brain: The Neural Basis of Mental Symptoms.* London: Gaskill.

Mayer-Gross, W., Slater, E. and Roth, M. (1954, 1960 and 1969) *Clinical Psychiatry,* 1st, 2nd and 3rd edns. London: Baillière, Tindall & Cassell.

Myers, D.G. and Diener, E. (1996) 'The pursuit of happiness: new research uncovers some anti-intuitive insights into how many people are happy – and why.' *Scientific American 274*, 54–56.

Negrete, J.C. (2000) In M. Gelder, J.J. López-Ibor and N.C. Andreasen (eds) *New Oxford Textbook of Psychiatry.* Oxford: Oxford University Press.

Pine-Coffin, R.S. (ed) (1961) *Saint Augustine: Confessions.* London: Penguin.

Ramachandran, V.S. (2003) *The Emerging Mind.* London: Profile Books.

Sims, A.C.P. (1993) 'Schizophrenia and permeability of self.' *Neurology, Psychiatry and Brain Research 1*, 133–155.

Sims, A. (2002) *Symptoms in the Mind,* 3rd edn. London: Saunders.

Sims, A. (2003) *Symptoms in the Mind: An Introduction to Descriptive Psychopathology,* 3rd edn. Edinburgh: Saunders.

Tolstoy, L. (1885) 'Where love is, God is.' In *Collected Shorter Fiction*, Volume 2. London: Everyman.

Tournier, P. (1963) *The Strong and the Weak*. Transl. E. Hudson. London: SCM Press.

Tournier, P. (1954) *A Doctor's Casebook in the Light of the Bible*. Transl. E. Hudson. London: SCM Press.

Uttal, W.R. (2001) *The New Phrenology: the Limits of Localizing Cognitive Processes in the Brain*. Cambridge, MA: MIT Press.

Ward, K. (1998) *God, Faith and the New Millenium: Christian Belief in an Age of Science*. Oxford: One World Publications.

World Health Organization (1992) *The ICD 10 Classification of Mental and Behavioural Disorders*. Geneva: World Health Organization.

BIBLIOGRAPHY OF BOOKS BY PAUL TOURNIER

Hans-Rudolf Pfeifer

FRENCH

The books here appear by date of first publication. The English titles of translated editions are included but note that the titles may not have been literal translations. Books have been numbered for ease of cross-referencing with the lists of English and German editions.

(1940) *Médecine de la Personne* [The Healing of Persons]. Neuchâtel, Switzerland: Delachaux et Niestlé. [1]

(1943) *De la Solitude à la Communauté* [Escape from Loneliness]. Neuchâtel, Switzerland: Delachaux et Niestlé. [2]

(1946) *Technique et Foi* [The Person Reborn]. Neuchâtel, Switzerland: Delachaux et Niestlé. [3]

(1947) *Désharmonie de la Vie Moderne* [The Whole Person in a Broken World]. Neuchâtel, Switzerland: Delachaux et Niestlé. [4]

(1948) *Les Forts et les Faibles* [The Strong and the Weak]. Neuchâtel, Switzerland: Delachaux et Niestlé. [5]

(1951) *Bible et Médecine* [A Doctor's Casebook in the Light of the Bible]. Neuchâtel, Switzerland: Delachaux et Niestlé. [6]

(1955) *Le Personnage et la Personne* [The Meaning of Persons]. Neuchâtel, Switzerland: Delachaux et Niestlé. [7]

(1958) *Vraie et Fausse Culpabilité* [Guilt and Grace]. Neuchâtel, Switzerland: Delachaux et Niestlé. [8]

(1961) *Des Cadeaux, Pourquoi?* [The Meaning of Gifts]. Geneva: Labor et Fides. [9]

(1961) *Les Saisons de la Vie* [The Seasons of Life]. Geneva: Labor et Fides. [10]

(1962) *Tenir Tête ou Céder* [To Resist or to Surrender]. Geneva: Labor et Fides. [11]

(1962) *Difficultés Conjugales* [To Understand Each Other]. Geneva: Labor et Fides. [12]

(1963) *Le Secret* [Secrets]. Geneva: Labor et Fides. [13]

(1963) *L'Aventure de la Vie* [The Adventure of Living]. Neuchâtel, Switzerland: Delachaux et Niestlé. [14]

(1966) *L'Homme et Son Lieu* [A Place for You]. Neuchâtel, Switzerland: Delachaux et Niestlé. [15]

(1971) *Apprendre à Vieillir* [Learn to Grow Old]. Neuchâtel, Switzerland: Delachaux et Niestlé. [16]

(1974) *Quel Nom lui Donnerez-Vous?* [What's in a Name?]. Geneva: Labor et Fides. [17]

(1977) *Violence et Puissance* [The Violence Within]. Neuchâtel, Switzerland: Delachaux et Niestlé. [18]

(1979) *La Mission de la Femme* [The Gift of Feeling]. Neuchâtel, Switzerland: Delachaux et Niestlé. [19]

(1981) *Face à la Souffrance* [Creative Suffering]. Geneva: Labor et Fides. [20]

(1984) *Vivre à l'Écoute* [A Listening Ear: Reflections on Christian Caring]. Editions de Caux. [21]

ENGLISH

The books here appear by date of first publication in English. Numerical indicators correspond with the respective French or German editions.

(1954) *A Doctor's Casebook in the Light of the Bible.* London: SCM Press. [6]

(1957) *The Meaning of Persons.* London: SCM Press. [7]

(1962) *Escape from Lonliness.* London: SCM Press. [2]

(1962) *Guilt and Grace.* London: Hodder and Stoughton. [8]

(1963) *The Strong and the Weak.* London: SCM Press. [5]

(1963) *The Meaning of Gifts.* Richmond, VA: John Knox. [9]

(1963) *The Seasons of Life.* Richmond, VA: John Knox. [10]

(1964) *The Whole Person in a Broken World.* London: SCM Press. [4]

(1964) *To Resist or to Surrender.* London: SCM Press. [11]

(1965) *The Healing of Persons.* London: Collins. [1]

(1965) *The Adventure of Living.* New York: Harpur and Row. [14]

(1965) *Secrets.* London: SCM Press. [13]

(1966) *The Person Reborn.* New York: Harpur and Row. [3]

(1967) *To Understand Each Other.* Richmond, VA: John Knox. [12]

(1968) *A Place for You.* London: SCM Press. [15]

(1972) *Learning to Grow Old.* London: SCM Press. [16]

(1975) *What's in a Name?* London: SCM Press. [17]

(1978) *The Violence Within.* London: SCM Press. [18]

(1981) *The Gift of Feeling.* Atlanta, GA: John Knox. [19]

(1982) *Creative Suffering.* London: SCM Press. [20]

(1986) *A Listening Ear: Fifty Years as a Doctor of the Whole Person.* Texts selected by Charles Piguet. Sevenoaks: Hodder and Stoughton. [21]

GERMAN

The books here appear by date of first publication. The English titles of translated editions are included where applicable but note that the titles may not have been literal translations. Books have been numbered for ease of cross-referencing with the lists of English and French editions.

(1941) *Krankheit und Lebensprobleme* [The Healing of Persons]. Basel: Schwabe & Co. [1]

(1944) *Aus der Vereinsamung zur Gemeinschaft* [Escape from Lonliness]. Basel: Schwabe & Co. [2]

(1945) *Technik und Glaube* [The Person Reborn]. Basel: Schwabe & Co. [3]

(1949) *Der Zwiespalt des modernen Menschen* [The Whole Person in Broken World]. Basel: Schwabe & Co. [4]

(1952) *Die Starken und die Schwachen* [The Strong and the Weak]. Basel: Schwabe & Co. [5]

(1953) *Bibel und Medizin* [A Doctor's Casebook in the Light of the Bible]. Zürich: Rascher. [6]

(1959) *Echtes und falsches Schuldgefühl* [Guilt and Grace]. Zürich: Rascher. [8]

(1961) *Unsere Maske und wir* [The Meaning of Persons]. Göttingen: Vandenhoeck & Ruprecht. [7]

(1961) *Geschenke und ihr Sinn* [The Meaning of Gifts]. Bern: Humata. [9]

(1962) *Sich durchsetzen und nachgeben* [To Resist or to Surrender]. Bern: Humata. [11]

(1963) *Leben, das grosse Abenteuer* [The Adventure of Living]. Bern: Humata. [14]

(1964) *Mehr Verständnis in der Ehe* [To Understand Each Other]. Bern: Humata. [12]

(1965) *Jeder hütet sein Geheimnis* [Secrets]. Zürich: Rascher. [13]

(1969) *Geborgenheit, Sehnsucht des Menschen* [A Place for You]. Bern: Humata. [15]

(1971) *Erfülltes Alter* [Learn to Grow Old]. Bern: Humata. [16]

(1977) *Die Jahreszeiten unseres Lebens* [The Seasons of Life]. Gütersloh: Gütersloher Verlagshaus. [10]

(1979) *Aggression, Kraft zum Guten, Kraft zum Bösen* [The Violence Within]. Zürich: Gotthelf. [17]

(1980) *Mutig Leben* [not translated]. Texts selected by Roche, Ch. de. Basel: Friedrich Reinhardt.

(1981) *Rückkehr zum Weiblichen* [The Gift of Feeling]. Freiburg: Herder. [18]

(1983) *Im Angesicht des Leidens* [Creative Suffering]. Freiburg: Herder. [19]

(1983) *Liebe gibt dem Leben Sinn* [not translated]. Texts selected by Roche, Ch. de. Basel: Friedrich Reinhardt.

(1986) *Zuhören können* [A Listening Ear: Reflections on Christian Caring]. Freiburg: Herder. [20]

(1987) *Antworten, die das Leben gibt* [not translated] Freiburg: Herder.

OTHER BOOKS RELATING TO PAUL TOURNIER

Collins, G.R. (1973) *The Christian Psychology of Paul Tournier.* Grand Rapids, MI: Baker Book House.

Harnick, B. (1972) *Risk and Chance in Marriage.* Foreword by Paul Tournier. Waco, TX: Word Books.

Harnick, B. (ed) (1973) *Paul Tournier's Medicine of the Whole Person.* Waco, TX: Word Books.

Lechler, W. (ed) (2004) *Die Schweigende Gegenwart – The Silent Presence – La Presence Silencieuse.* Geesthacht: Neuland Verlag.

Peaston, M. (1972) *Personal Living – An Introduction to Paul Tournier.* New York: Harper and Row.

Roche, Ch. de. and Reinhardt, E. (1987) *Paul Tournier, ein Leben – eine Botschaft* [not translated]. Basel: Friedrich Reinhardt.

Tournier, P. (ed) (1965) *Fatigue in Modern Society.* Richmond, VA: John Knox Press.

Tournier, P. (1976) *A Tournier Companion.* London: SCM Press.

Tournier, P., Frankl, V., Levinson, H. and Thielicke, H. (1966) 'The Person in an Age of Conformity.' In K. Haselden (ed) *Are You Nobody?* Richmond, VA: John Knox Press.

THESES ON PAUL TOURNIER

Bindschedler, J.D. (1954). *Le Fondement Théologique de la Médecine de la Personne.* Thèse, Université de Strasbourg, Faculté de Théologie Protestante.

Clark, J. (1974) *The Contribution of Paul Tournier to Christian Education and Guidance in Schools.* Unpublished PhD Thesis, University of Exeter.

Hagner, B.S (1980). 'Values in psychotherapy: a study of the presence and impact of value assumptions in the counselling process.' *Dissertation Abstracts International 41,* 1108B. University Microfilms No. 80-20, 659.

Houde, K.A. (1990). *The Christian Personality Theory of Paul Tournier.* Doctoral dissertation, Fuller Theological Seminary.

McKain, W.H., Jr (1978). 'The contributions of Paul Tournier to the practice of pastoral counselling.' *Dissertation Abstracts International 39,* 2367A. University Microfilms No. 78-18, 602.

Pfeifer, H.-R. (1994). *Personzentrierte und sinnorientierte existentielle Psychotherapie. Eine vergleichende Studie über Leben und Werk von Paul Tournier (Médecine de la Personne) und Viktor E.Frankl (Logotherapie und Existenzanalyse).* Medizinische Fakultät Basel.

Rynbrandt, T.P. (1971). *An Evaluation of the Concept of Guilt in Selected Writings of Paul Tournier.* Ph.D dissertation, Fuller Theological Seminary.

LIST OF CONTRIBUTORS

Robert Atwell is an Anglican priest. After six years as Chaplain of Trinity College, Cambridge, where he taught Patristics, he became a Benedictine monk, spending the next ten years in a monastery in the Cotswolds. He is the compiler of two volumes of daily readings for the liturgical year, *Celebrating the Saints* and *Celebrating the Seasons*, and of three anthologies of readings, *Love, Gift* and *Remember*. He is currently vicar of the parish of St Mary the Virgin, Primrose Hill, London.

Dinesh Bhugra is currently Professor of Mental Health and Cultural Diversity at the Institute of Psychiatry, King's College, London and honorary consultant at the Maudsley Hospital. He trained in psychiatry, anthropology and sociology after graduating in medicine from Pune University. His research interests include cross-cultural psychiatry, spirituality and psychosexual dysfunction. He is the editor of *International Review of Psychiatry* and *International Journal of Social Psychiatry* and has published several books, including *Religion and Psychiatry* and the monograph *Mad Tales from Bollywood*.

Alastair V. Campbell is the Chen Su Lan Centennial Professor of Medical Ethics at the medical school of the National University of Singapore. He was formerly Director of the Centre for Ethics in Medicine at University of Bristol. He is a former President of the International Association of Bioethics. Recent publications include *Health as Liberation* (Pilgrim Press, 1995) and *Medical Ethics*, 4th edn, co-authored with Grant Gillett and Gareth Jones (Oxford University Press, 2005). Professor Campbell is a member of the Medical Ethics Committee of the British Medical Association. Until recently, Professor Campbell was Chairman of the Wellcome Trust's Standing Advisory Group on Ethics and Vice-chairman of the Retained Organs Commission. He is currently Chairman of the UK Biobank's Ethics and Governance Council.

John Clark studied History and Theology at Oxford University and is a Licensed Lay Reader in the Anglican Church. Before retirement, he was the Director of Studies in a large school and a College Senior Lecturer in Student Guidance. John found Tournier's work highly relevant after first reading *The Meaning of Persons*. He met Tournier on several occasions and wrote a Doctoral thesis at Exeter University on 'The Contribution of Paul Tournier to Christian Education'. He is a longstanding member of the British and International Medicine of the Person Groups.

Thierry Collaud studied medicine, philosophy and theology in Switzerland and United States. He works part time as a general practitioner in Neuchâtel, Switzerland and part time as a theologian in the department of Catholic Moral Theology of the University of Fribourg, Switzerland. He had published in 2003 *Le Statut de la Personne Démente. Éléments d'une Anthropologie de l'Homme Malade* (Academic Press, Fribourg).

Martin Conway has had a career stretching from the staff of the Student Christian Movement to serving as President of the Selly Oak Colleges in Birmingham and as simultaneous interpreter at successive Assemblies of the World Council of Churches. He is a lay member of the Church of England and Chairman of the Oxford Diocesan Board for Social Responsibility.

John Cox studied Medicine at Oxford University, and Psychiatry in London. He is currently Secretary General of the World Psychiatric Association and Professor Emeritus at Keele University, Staffordshire. He is a Past President of the Royal College of Psychiatrists and has published extensively in perinatal mental health. He retains his interest in transcultural psychiatry and in the boundaries of religion and mental health. He lives in the Lake District.

Tom Fryers MD PhD FFPH trained in Manchester and specialised in Public Health in Salford before teaching at Manchester Medical School for over 20 years. For over 40 years he has been involved in research and development in mental health and disability, working in many countries, including Nigeria, Zambia, Mauritius, China, and Bosnia. Currently he is Visiting Professor of Public Mental Health, Leicester University, and Visiting Lecturer in International Health, New York Medical College, and is a Methodist Local Preacher.

Bill (K.W.M.) Fulford is Professor of Philosophy and Mental Health in the Department of Philosophy and the Medical School, University of Warwick; an Honorary Consultant Psychiatrist in the Department of Psychiatry, University of Oxford; and Special Professional Adviser for Values- Based Practice to the Care Services Directorate and the Care Services Improvement Partnership in the Department of Health, London. He is also the Founder and Editor of *Philosophy, Psychiatry and Psychology*.

Peter Gilbert is Professor of Social Work and Spirituality at Staffordshire University and NIMHE Lead on the national 'Spirituality and Mental Health' Project. A social worker by background, Peter was Director of Social Services for Worcestershire, and is the author of *Leadership: Being Effective and Remaining Human*. A co-facilitator of retreats for busy professionals at Worth Abbey, Peter is currently co-editing a book on spirituality and mental health for Jessica Kingsley Publishers.

Michael Hilton is Rabbi of Kol Chai Hatch End Jewish Community in the London Borough of Harrow. He is an Honorary Research Fellow of the Centre for Jewish Studies at Manchester University and the author of *The Christian Effect on Jewish Life* (1994, London: SCM).

Claire Hilton is a Consultant Psychiatrist for older people in the London Borough of Harrow at the Central and North West London Mental Health NHS Trust.

Mike Magee is Senior Research Fellow in the Humanities to the World Medical Association, Director of the Pfizer Medical Humanities Initiative and host of the popular Internet programme 'Health Politics with Dr Mike Magee'. He is the author of several books and writes and speaks frequently on a wide range of health policy issues.

Ahmed Okasha is Professor and Director of the World Health Organization Collaborating Center for Training and Research in Mental Health, Institute of Psychiatry, Ain Shams University, Cairo, and is President of the Egyptian Psychiatric Association, Immediate Past President of the World Psychiatric Association and member of the Advisory Council of the World Psychiatric Association.

Hans-Rudolf Pfeifer is a psychiatrist and psychotherapist, Head of a psychiatric clinic in Zurich Canton, Switzerland. He is also a founding member of the Paul Tournier Association in Troinex, Geneva. His doctoral thesis was on Paul Tournier (Médicine de la Personne) and Victor E. Frankl (Existential Analysis and Logotherapy). He is President of the Christian Medical fellowship of Switzwerland (AGEAS). He is married and has two children.

Bernard Rüedi is Chairman Emeritus of the Department of Internal Medicine, City Hospital, Neuchâtel, Switzerland and was Associate Professor of Endocrinology, University of Lausanne and Professor of Medical Psychology, University of Neuchâtel. He is Past President of the Swiss Society of Internal Medicine and Past President of the Swiss Society of Medical Informatics. Bernard is a long-standing member of the International Group of Medicine of the Person.

Andrew Sims is Emeritus Professor of Psychiatry, University of Leeds and Past President, Royal College of Psychiatrists. He chaired the Spirituality and Psychiatry Special Interest Group of the Royal College 2003–2005. His interests include the epidemiology and outcome studies in non-psychotic psychiatric conditions, descriptive psychopathology and the interface between religious experience and psychiatric symptoms. He is the author of *Symptoms in the Mind* (three editions), and other books and journal articles.

SUBJECT INDEX

abortion 84–5, 89–90
addiction 213–15
Africa 74, 98
Age Concern 152
alcoholism 213–15
Alzheimer's disease 193, 200
Anglicanism 84–5, 89, 150
anxiety 176, 177, 183
  care-givers 192, 193
Arabic cultures 112–14
  cognitive style 112–14
  decision-making 117–18
  dependence versus
    independence
    116–17
  gender 118–19, 120–2
  individualism 116
  Islam 114–15
  language 114
  mental illness 118–20,
    121
  social and family systems
    115–16, 122–3
Asia 98
atheism 41
Ayurvedic tradition 125,
  133–5, 136, 137

Barth, Karl 165
behaviourism 125
Benedict XVI 141
Benedictine Abbey, Worth,
  Sussex 147–8
Bennett, David 149
Bennett, Dr Joanna 149
Bible 13–14, 22–3, 40,
  56–7
  biblical themes 57–8,
    214, 221
  grace and growth 58–9
  guilt and reconciliation
    59–60

medical practice 60–3
  values 79–80
biological effect 51
Bordes, Jan de 37
Bosnia 186
Bovet, Theo 39
brain function 122–3,
  208–9, 218
Breath of Life 150
British Medical Journal 25
British Psychological
  Association 150
Brunner, Emil 18, 36, 57
Buchmann, Frank 37
Buddhism 41, 49, 67, 75,
  76, 110

Calvinism 33, 36, 83
Camberwell Family
  Interview 119
care 175–7
  care-givers 192–5, 201
  dependence 179–80
  elderly people 190–3
  home-based 200–5
  interdependence 177–8
  see also person-centred
    care
caste 132, 133
cause and effect 211–12
centenarians 190
children 72–3, 179
China 76
Christianity 9, 13, 14, 18,
  24, 41, 75, 175,
  207–8, 216, 217, 221,
  222
  community development
    185–7
  death 63
  guilt 59–60
  healing 93–4
  interdependence 177–8,
    182–3
  Paul Tournier 22–3, 27,
    48–9, 59, 65–8
  spirituality 172–3, 174,
    219–20
  values 79–80

Church of England 84–5,
  89, 150
community 24, 25, 26,
  185–7
  Arabic cultures 116
  individualism 173–5
  Judaism 100–2
Community Security Trust
  98
compunction 90–1
Confucianism 76, 110
consequentialism 21
counselling 84–5
  non-directive counselling
    22, 25
  pastoral counselling 25,
    84–5, 90, 120
  spiritual direction 85–6
cremation 106
crises 91
criticism 65, 118–19
cultural identities 111–12

death 63, 107
  end of life care 196–200
dependency 176–7, 182–3,
  184–5
depression 51, 118–19,
  176, 183
  care-givers 192, 193,
    201
  local government
    employment 146–7
  prevalence 176, 177
Desert Fathers and Mothers
  23, 87, 89
desires 91–2
disabled people 176
discernment, process of 85,
  92–4
doctor–patient relationship
  19–20, 24, 25, 26, 27,
  219
  elderly care 193–6
  expectations 46–7
  medicine of the person
    94–5
  reciprocity 49

AUTHOR INDEX